Advances in Gerontological Nursing

1996
Issues for The 21st Century
Elizabeth A. Swanson, PhD, RN, and
Toni Tripp-Reimer, PhD, RN, FAAN, Editors

1997
Chronic Illness and the Older Adults
Elizabeth A. Swanson, PhD, RN, and
Toni Tripp-Reimer, PhD, RN, FAAN, Editors

1999
Life Transitions in the Older Adult:
Issues for Nurses and Other Health Professionals
Elizabeth A. Swanson, PhD, RN, and
Toni Tripp-Reimer, PhD, RN, FAAN, Editors

Elizabeth A. Swanson, Ph.D., R.N., is an Associate Professor in the College of Nursing at The University of Iowa, in Iowa City, Iowa. Dr. Swanson received a B.S. in nursing and an M.A. from The University of Iowa College of Nursing, as well as a Ph.D. from the College of Education.

Her work focuses on examining the effects of the nursing interventions of family-staff partnerships on staff, family, and residents diagnosed with Alzheimer's disease. She also is involved in research projects that investigate the impact of individualized music therapy and group music therapy on persons with Alzheimer's disease and dementia.

Toni Tripp-Reimer, Ph.D., R.N., F.A.A.N., is Professor and Associate Dean for Research at The University of Iowa College of Nursing in Iowa City, Iowa. Dr. Tripp-Reimer received a B.S.N. from the University of Maryland. She holds an M.S. in nursing and an M.A. and Ph.D. in anthropology from The Ohio State University. She also is Director (or PI) of the NIH-funded Center for Gerontological Nursing Interventions Research (P30), the Institutional NRSA Training Program in Gerontological Nursing Research (T32), and the Iowa-Veterans Affairs Nursing Research Consortium.

She has conducted work concerned with health behaviors of ethnic older persons for the past 18 years through a series of seven funded projects. Her current work focuses on issues of medication self-care for rural older adults, psychosocial issues in relocation, and assessment and management of acute confusion.

Life Transitions in the Older Adult

Issues for Nurses and Other Health Professionals

Elizabeth Swanson, PhD, RN
Toni Tripp-Reimer, PhD, RN, FAAN
Editors

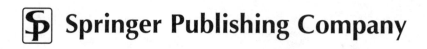 Springer Publishing Company

Springer Publishing Company, Inc.
536 Broadway
New York, NY 10012–3955

Cover design by Janet Joachim
Acquisitions Editor: Ruth Chasek
Production Editor: Jeanne Libby

99 00 01 02 03 / 5 4 3 2 1

ISBN 0-8261-9112-6
ISSN 1083-8708

Printed in the United States of America

Contents

Contributors

Barbara M. Barer, M.S.W.
Medical Anthropology Program
University of California, San Francisco
San Francisco, California 94143-0850
e-mail: bbarer@gateway.net

Perle Slavik Cowen, R.N., Ph.D.
Assistant Professor
College of Nursing
The University of Iowa
Iowa City, Iowa 52242
e-mail: perle-cowen@uiowa.edu

Lorraine T. Dorfman, Ph.D.
Professor
School of Social Work
Director, Aging Studies Program
The University of Iowa
Iowa City, Iowa 52242
e-mail: lorraine-dorfman@uiowa.edu

Colleen L. Johnson, Ph.D.
Medical Anthropology Program
University of California, San Francisco
San Francisco, California 94143-0850
e-mail: cljoo@itsa.ucsf.edu

Rebecca A. Johnson, Ph.D., R.N.
Assistant Professor
School of Nursing
Northern Illinois University
DeKalb, Illinois 60115
e-mail: r60rajl@wpo.cso.niu.edu

Patricia S. Jones, R.N., Ph.D.
Professor
Adult and Aging Family Nursing
School of Nursing
Loma Linda University
Loma Linda, California 92350
e-mail: jones_patricia@ccmail.llumc.edu

David L. Kahn, Ph.D., R.N.
Assistant Professor
School of Nursing
University of Texas at Austin
Austin, Texas 78759
e-mail: dkahn@mail.utexas.edu

Meridean L. Maas, Ph.D., R.N., F.A.A.N.
Professor
College of Nursing
The University of Iowa
Iowa City, Iowa 52242
e-mail: meridean-maas@uiowa.edu

Afaf Ibrahim Meleis, Ph.D., Dr.P.S. (hon), F.A.A.N.
Professor
Department of Community Health Systems
School of Nursing
University of California, San Francisco
San Francisco, California 94143-0608
e-mail: meleis@itsa.ucsf.edu

Janet C. Mentes, R.N.C.S., M.S.
Predoctoral Fellow and Research Assistant
College of Nursing
The University of Iowa
Iowa City, Iowa 52242
e-mail: janet-mentes@uiowa.edu

Carla Gene Rapp, M.N.Sc., R.N., C.R.R.N.
Predoctoral Fellow and Research Assistant
College of Nursing
The University of Iowa
Iowa City, Iowa 52242
e-mail: carla-rapp@uiowa.edu

David Reed, Ph.D.
Research Project Director
College of Nursing
The University of Iowa
Iowa City, Iowa 52242
e-mail: david-reed@uiowa.edu

Patricia T. Riley, B.S.N., R.N.
Graduate Research Assistant
College of Nursing
The University of Iowa
Iowa City, Iowa 52242
e-mail: patricia-riley@uiowa.edu

Karen L. Schumacher, Ph.D., R.N.
Assistant Adjunct Professor
Department of Community Health Systems
School of Nursing
University of California, San Francisco
San Francisco, California 94143
e-mail: Karen_schumacher_at_nursing@ccmail.ucsf.edu

Debra Schutte, M.S.N., R.N.
Program Assistant
College of Nursing
The University of Iowa
Iowa City, Iowa 52242
e-mail: debra-schutte@uiowa.edu

Lisa Skemp-Kelley, M.S.N, R.N.
Program Assistant
College of Nursing
The University of Iowa
Iowa City, Iowa 52242
e-mail: lisa-kelley@uiowa.edu

Janet P. Specht, Ph.D., R.N.
Research Scientist
College of Nursing
The University of Iowa
Iowa City, Iowa 52242
e-mail: janet-specht@uiowa.edu

Richard H. Steeves, Ph.D., R.N., F.A.A.N.
Associate Professor
School of Nursing
University of Virginia
Charlottesville, Virginia 22908
e-mail: rhs2p@virginia.edu

Kay Weiler, R.N., M.A., J.D.
Associate Professor
College of Nursing
The University of Iowa
Iowa City, Iowa 52242
e-mail: kay-weiler@uiowa.edu

National Advisory Panel

Ivo L. Abraham, Ph.D., C.S., R.N., F.A.A.N.
Professor
Schools of Nursing and Medicine
Charlottesville, Virginia 22903
and
Catholic University of Leuven
Leuven, Belgium

Patricia G. Archbold, R.N., D.N.Sc., F.A.A.N.
Professor
School of Nursing
Oregon Health Sciences University
Portland, Oregon 97201

Cornelia M. Beck, Ph.D., R.N., F.A.A.N.
Professor and Associate Dean for Research and Evaluation
College of Nursing
University of Arkansas for Medical Sciences
Little Rock, Arkansas 72205

Barbara A. Given, Ph.D., R.N., F.A.A.N.
Professor and Director of Research
College of Nursing
Michigan State University
East Lansing, Michigan 48824

Virgene Kayser-Jones, Ph.D., R.N., F.A.A.N.
Professor
School of Nursing
University of California-San Francisco
San Francisco, California 94143

Kathleen A. McCormick, Ph.D., R.N., F.A.A.N.
Senior Science Advisor
Office of Science and Data Development
Agency for Health Care Policy and Research
Rockville, Maryland 20852

Virginia J. Neelon, Ph.D., R.N.
Associate Professor and Director
Biobehavioral Laboratory
School of Nursing
The University of North Carolina at Chapel Hill
Chapel Hill, North Carolina 27599

Linda R. Phillips, Ph.D., R.N., F.A.A.N.
Professor
College of Nursing
University of Arizona
Tucson, Arizona 85721

Neville E. Strumpf, Ph.D., R.N., C., F.A.A.N.
Associate Professor
School of Nursing
University of Pennsylvania
Philadelphia, Pennsylvania 19104

Thelma J. Wells, Ph.D., R.N., F.A.A.N., F.R.C.N.
Professor
School of Nursing
University of Wisconsin
Madison, Wisconsin 53792

May L. Wykle, Ph.D., R.N., F.A.A.N.
Florence Cellar Professor and Chairperson of Gerontological Nursing
FPB School of Nursing
Case Western Reserve University
Cleveland, Ohio 44106

Introduction

This volume focuses on the impact of transition on elderly persons—particularly on their health and sense of well-being. Transitions are defined as passages from one state, stage, subject, or place to another. In the following chapters, the authors define transition within the context of health, role relationships, expectations, and abilities. They classify transitions into different stages: familial transitions, health/illness transitions, individual transitions, and circumstantial transitions. We believe that gerontological nurses, in collaboration with other health professionals, are in a significant position to promote the well-being of older adults in periods of transition. It is hoped that gerontological nurses, researchers, and other health professionals will use the information provided in this volume to formulate interventions and strategies to facilitate positive transitions and minimize health risks for older adults.

In the opening chapter, "Helping Elderly Persons in Transition: A Framework for Practice," Schumacher, Jones, and Meleis lay a firm foundation for the volume by proposing a theoretical framework for transition that is useful both in practice and research. The authors discuss the many transitions experienced by older adults, review conceptual work and nursing research on transitions, and identify characteristics and indicators of healthy transitions. In closing, the authors describe several nursing interventions to assist with the transition process and demonstrate the applicability of the framework through the use of a case study. Echoes of many of the conceptual elements introduced by Schumacher, Jones, and Meleis can be heard in several of the subsequent chapters of this volume.

In the second chapter, "Retirement: Health Issues, Perspectives, and Policy Considerations," Dorfman and Rapp discuss what they view as the major transition of later life for older persons living in industrialized societies. The authors present recent research on the effects of health on retirement, the effects of retirement on health, and the association between health and retirement adjustment. They conclude that the most important role of the nurse in working with older adults who retire is to provide information and educate the prospective retirees. In using this knowledge, practitioners and researchers can assist older adults to achieve a healthier outcome.

The next chapters focus on caregiving for older family members during certain transitional phases: residential caregiving, institutional placement, and bereavement. As previously noted, there is often a series of changes within the transitional period that places demands on caregivers and has an effect on the activities and roles they undertake and the manner in which they perceive themselves. To truly assist in these transitional phases, gerontological nurses need to be aware of the effect of extended caregiving on family members and the care recipients.

Johnson in chapter 3, "Helping Older Adults Adjust to Relocation," supports the role of nursing in assisting persons in transition, particularly to a nursing home. She presents the research from the past 20 years related to relocation and focuses the discussion on the empirically based interventions that can help persons adjust positively in this relocation process. Similarly, relocations of residents within a long-term-care facility are a fairly common event. In chapter 4, "Relocating Elderly Persons with Dementia," Specht and her colleagues examine the effects of relocation on older adults, reasons for relocation, and the effects of relocation on Special Care Unit residents and their families. The authors suggest strategies to promote the healthy relocation of older persons with dementia.

As Steeves and Kahn acknowledge in chapter 5, "Coping with Death," loss is a part of aging. After discussing what is known about bereavement and its effects on older adults, they identify the factors that influence the trajectory of bereavement and review interventions that have been evaluated for their efficacy in the older population. In closing, Steeves and Kahn suggest an intervention composed of three tasks that are crucial for the bereaved to complete prior to putting their lives in order.

Chapters 6 and 7 of this volume focus on a transitional experience that could be defined as circumstantial in nature: contemporary grandparenting. Grandparents in some cases are being placed in ambiguous circumstances caused by divorces of their children, while in others they are assuming the roles of surrogate parents or custodial parents. In "Grandparents in the Contemporary Family," Johnson and Barer examine how grandparents define their role and how the structure and functioning of grandparenting changes, often with ambiguous results, with divorce. Then

Mentes, in "Cultural Aspects of Grandparents Raising Grandchildren," considers the effect of race on grandparenting when looking at intergenerational family issues of family structure and kinship relations. From their distinct perspectives, these authors help shed light on the critical issues of who benefits from the caregiving arrangements, the effect of ethnicity, and what issues gerontological nurses need to be aware of when grandparents become the caregivers of their grandchildren.

In chapter 8, "Legal and Ethical Issues for Older Adults," Weiler and Slavik Cowen offer another perspective on the experiences of older adults in a period of transition. The authors note that many of the changes associated with aging entail legal and ethical issues that older adults and those caring for them must consider. To examine those critical issues, the authors focus on the four principles of autonomy, beneficence, nonmaleficence, and justice. The provision of this information through the four principles is similar to what Schumacher and her colleagues describe as the developing of new knowledge and skills and the creating of new options: both are indicators of a healthy transition process. Weiler and Slavik Cowen conclude their chapter with what we define as a most dire consequence of an unhealthy transition—mistreatment of older adults.

Whether the transition is circumstantial, familial, or individual, our contributors to this volume all acknowledge the stressful conditions that are created for older adults and their family members. With this acknowledgment comes the responsibility that gerontological nurses critically assess the situation and intervene appropriately to lessen the degree of adverse effects on the elderly and facilitate their adjustment. It is through this comprehensive assessment that nurses can intervene in the practice and/or policy arena. In addition, it is crucial that educators and scholars use this information to inform students and to develop theoretically derived research programs to examine the positive and negative effects of transitional phases of life. Transitions should not be viewed as just another aspect of growing old.

CHAPTER 1

Helping Elderly Persons in Transition: A Framework for Research and Practice

Karen L. Schumacher, Patricia S. Jones, and Afaf Ibrahim Meleis

G rowing old is not an event. There is not a particular day or a certain birthday that marks a person as old. Growing old is a process of gains and losses that takes time. How this period of time is viewed by gerontological nurses shapes their work with elderly clients and their families. The nature of nursing assessment, the goals established with clients, and the interventions used are embedded in the nurse's perspective on aging. Similarly, the research questions posed by the gerontological nurse are embedded in a particular perspective.

We propose that a transition framework provides a perspective on aging with significant potential for advancing gerontological nursing practice and research. Many transitions are experienced by elderly persons, and these transitions are inherently linked to the older person's health and need for nursing care. Indeed, it often is a transition that brings the older person into contact with professional nursing. The use of a transition framework recognizes the importance of transitions for the health of elderly persons. Thus such a perspective leads to effective strategies for practice and productive lines of inquiry for research.

The purpose of this chapter is to describe a transition framework for use in gerontological nursing practice and research and to demonstrate its use.

We first provide an overview of transitions in elderly persons, briefly reviewing both conceptual work and nursing research on transitions. Next, we turn our attention to transitions and health, identifying characteristics and indicators of healthy transition processes. Finally, we describe several nursing therapeutics designed to facilitate smooth transitions for older clients. The use of this framework is demonstrated with a case example.

THE CONCEPT OF TRANSITION: DEFINITION AND PROPERTIES

A transition is a passage between two relatively stable periods of time. In this passage, the individual moves from one life phase, situation, or status to another. Transitions are processes that occur over time and have a sense of flow and movement. They are ushered in by changes that trigger a period of disequilibrium and upheaval. During this period, the individual experiences profound changes in his or her external world and in the manner that world is perceived. There often is a sense of loss or of alienation from what had been familiar and valued. During transitions, new skills, new relationships, and new coping strategies need to be developed (Chick & Meleis, 1986; Meleis, 1986; Meleis & Trangenstein, 1994).

Late life is a time of multiple transitions. Retirement, loss of spouse and friends, relocation to a new living situation, and the advent of chronic illness or frailty are just some of the transitions experienced by elderly persons. These transitions may be categorized as developmental, situational, or related to health and illness (Figure 1.1). Many of the transitions experienced by older persons involve loss and are undesired. However, some transitions are positive and welcomed. For example, starting a new endeavor or developing new aspects of self are transitions that represent opportunities rather than losses.

What are the properties of a transition? First, a transition is precipitated by a significant marker event or turning point that requires new patterns of response. These markers prompt the recognition that business is not as usual and that new strategies are needed to handle even familiar, daily life experiences, such as managing one's finances, maintaining one's own health, or taking care of daily activities. Such strategies involve the development of new skills, new relationships, and new roles. Another characteristic of transitions is that they are processes that take time. Transitions span the whole period of time from the initial marker event until harmony

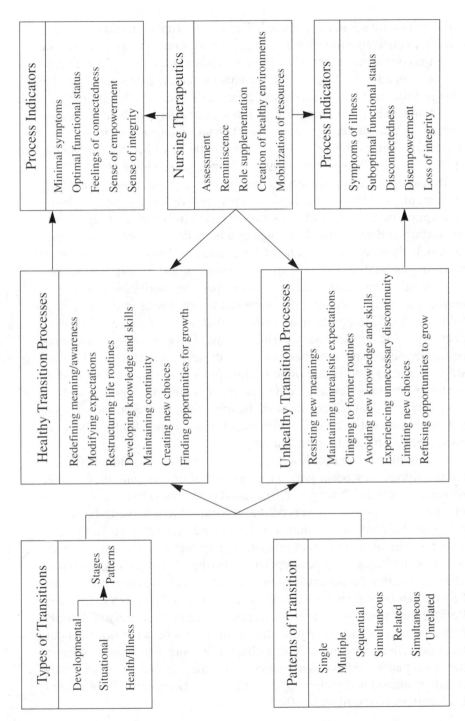

Figure 1.1 Transitions and health: A framework for gerontological nursing.

and stability are again experienced. This time period is needed to experiment with different strategies and patterns of responses and to incorporate them into one's own repertoire. The time required for a transition is variable and depends on the nature of the change and the extent to which that change influences other aspects of a person's life. Another property of transition is that changes in identity, roles, and patterns of behavior occur. Transitions are not fleeting or superficial changes; rather, they involve fundamental changes in one's view of self and the world (Chick & Meleis, 1986; Meleis & Trangenstein, 1994; Schumacher & Meleis, 1994).

Transitions often are conceptualized in terms of stages to capture their movement, direction, and flow as they evolve over time. A classic description of the stages of transition is found in Bridges' study (1980). According to Bridges, the first stage of a transition is a period of endings in which there is disengagement from relationships or from ways of behaving as well as a change in the person's sense of self. The second stage, termed the "neutral zone," is an in-between period, a time when a person experiences disorientation caused by the losses in the first stage followed by disintegration of systems that were in place. This is an uncomfortable but necessary period of time. Only by going through the neutral zone can persons become open to new possibilities. The final stage of a transition is that of new beginnings and is marked by finding meaning and experiencing some control. Persons must go through all three stages to deal effectively with the transition. However, the stages of a transition do not necessarily occur in a linear manner. Rather, they may be sequential, parallel, or overlapping.

Transitions also can be described in terms of patterns. Single or multiple transitions may occur within a given period of time, and they may be related or unrelated. Young (1990) alluded to the phenomenon of patterns of transition when she observed that relocation to a nursing home can occur in the context of other transitions and can catalyze further life changes. She also noted that relocation may include elements of situational, health/illness, and developmental transitions. Gerontological nurses often deal with such patterns of transition in clinical practice, but very little work has been done with theory development and research in this area. Fruitful directions for future scholarship would be to name and describe transition patterns and to explore the relationships between different patterns and client outcomes. In this chapter, we suggest three patterns of transition that we believe merit attention: (1) the sequential pattern, (2) the simultaneous/related pattern, and (3) the simultaneous/unrelated pattern. Each pattern is described briefly.

In sequential transitions, there is a ripple effect in which one transition leads to another over time. For example, the death of one's spouse may lead to relocation to a nursing home, or retirement from paid employment may lead to the emergence of new dimensions of self. It is possible for this ripple effect to extend over a long period of time. The instance in which retirement leads to insufficient income, which in turn leads to a decline in health status and eventually to chronic illness and loss of social interaction, is an example of a long-term, cumulative ripple effect.

Simultaneous transitions are clusters of related or unrelated transitions that occur together during a given period of time. In simultaneous, related transitions, a marker event precipitates numerous transitions. For example, the marker event of a stroke may usher in a cluster of transitions in functional abilities, identity, and living arrangements. The complexity of such transitions may be compounded by simultaneous transitions for the older adult's family members, who may take on the caregiving role and undergo changes in work and family roles. Ade-Ridder and Kaplan (1993) alluded to this pattern of transition when they noted that a transition for an older adult creates a variety of countertransitions for the family.

Simultaneous transitions also may occur without being initially related to one another. For example, an older adult may suffer a decline in health at the same time his or her adult child is experiencing the transition to an "empty nest." Such transitions in a given family happen concurrently and, although not directly related at first, may become intertwined over time.

NURSING RESEARCH ON TRANSITIONS

What has nursing research shown about transitions? First, transitions may be accompanied by uncertainty, emotional distress, interpersonal conflict, and worry. Michels (1988) documented the uncertainty experienced by family caregivers of elderly persons during the transition from hospital to home. Johnson, Morton, and Knox (1992) found that nursing home admissions, too, are characterized by uncertainty. In this transition, uncertainty was related to lack of information and knowledge about the nature of nursing homes and the boundaries for family involvement there. Families also described feelings of sadness and anger, as well as a sense of failure when an older adult was admitted to a nursing home. Lack of communication with nursing home staff added to the emotional conflict. The transition to needing assistance with self-care activities also may bring about emotional distress. For example, Conn, Taylor, and Messina (1995) investigated the transition to needing medication assistance and found that some older adults were frustrated, depressed, or angry about requiring assistance. The researchers noted that nurses should expect some caregivers and care recipients to experience difficulties in their relationship as the caregiver begins assisting the older adult and that they should be encouraged to express their feelings about these transitions in role relationships.

Bull (1992) found that the transition from hospital to home was characterized by worry. In semistructured interviews, participants identified worries ranging from apprehension about learning new skills to distress about disruption in the family's usual activities of daily living. Bull also described the movement from worry to mastery as the transition evolved. By 2 months after discharge from the hospital, participants had established new routines and felt in control of the situation. The movement from worry to mastery found in the interviews was corroborated by quantitative data that showed a steady decline in anxiety and depression (Bull, Maruyama, & Luo, 1995).

The study by Bull and colleagues (Bull, 1992; Bull, Maruyama, et al., 1995) is noteworthy for the way in which the dimension of time was incorporated into the research design. In this study, change over time was documented by collecting data at two points in the transition. Such a design is congruent with the nature of the transition experience. Because transitions are processes, research designs need to be planned so that they capture the evolution of the transition experience.

There is some evidence that older persons and their family members do not always receive the professional support they need during a transition. In Michel's (1988) study, 73% of the older adults returned to their homes with a home care regimen consisting of three or more components, such as prescription medications, dietary changes, assessment of signs and symptoms, and continuing care of an incision, tube, drain, or colostomy. Nearly two thirds had been instructed on how to care for themselves and carry out their prescribed regimen, but only half acknowledged that someone had asked if they had questions or concerns about their care before the transition to home took place. Some family members had difficulties assuming caregiving responsibilities, and they did not always have the opportunity to participate in discharge planning to prepare them for the transition. Bull, Jervis, and Her (1995) also found that some family members of older patients were inadequately prepared for hospital discharge, did not have the opportunity for input into discharge decisions, and encountered problems with the coordination of services. Stewart, Archbold,

Harvath, and Nkongho (1993) investigated a broad range of learning needs of family caregivers and found that health professionals were perceived as sources of information about taking care of the physical needs of the care receiver and setting up services in the home, but that caregivers reported learning very little from health professionals about taking care of the care receiver's emotional needs and handling the stress of caregiving.

TRANSITIONS AND HEALTH

We turn now to a consideration of transitions and health. What are the characteristics of a healthy transition? We approach this question by considering transition processes and process indicators (see Figure 1.1). Transition processes are the cognitive, behavioral, and interpersonal processes through which the transition unfolds. In other words, they are what happens during a transition. In healthy transitions, these processes move the individual in the direction of health, whereas in unhealthy transitions, they move the individual in the direction of vulnerability and risk.

Process indicators are measurable indices of how the transition is going at any point in time. A process indicator can be thought of as a stop-action snapshot of client well-being at a key point in the ongoing transition process. Assessed periodically, process indicators provide a way of tracking client progress through the transition. We use the term "process indicators" rather than "outcomes" because the process should be assessed periodically over the course of the transition, not just at its conclusion. When the older adult's experience is analyzed using a transition perspective, it is difficult to consider outcomes in the same way as when the older adult's experiences are viewed in isolation from time and significant others. From a transition perspective, "outcomes" evolve over the course of the transition and also are connected to life experiences prior to and after the transition. Process indicators could be used as client outcomes in research, but only with the caveat that they are part of the client's ongoing life experiences.

Healthy Transition Processes

Seven healthy transition processes and seven corresponding unhealthy processes are identified (see Figure 1.1). Over the course of the transition, there is a dynamic tension between healthy and unhealthy processes. Both the future toward which the transition is moving and the past that is being left behind exert a pull on the elderly client. These processes move the client through the "neutral zone" of the transition toward the next phase or situation in his or her life. The gerontological nurse should be alert to the presence of these processes in clients in transition and should monitor the direction in which they are proceeding.

1. Redefining meanings is one process that takes place during a healthy transition (Davis & Grant, 1994; Langner, 1995). The elderly client and his or her family actively engage in exploring the meaning of the transition and in finding new meanings. Previous meanings that do not apply to the new situation are recognized, and new meanings are discovered. The process of creating meaning is complex, and time is needed for the older person to work through it. When the transition is proceeding in a healthy direction, the general movement is toward rethinking and redefining meanings. In unhealthy transitions, there is resistance to redefining meanings. The older person and his or her family do not consider the meaning of the transition and attempt to apply old definitions to the new situation.

2. Modifying expectations is another process that characterizes healthy transitions. Long-standing expectations about self, others, and the future may be called into question during a transition (Dewar & Morse, 1995; King, Porter, & Rowe, 1994; Wilson & Billones, 1994), and the older person may be reluctant to give up these expectations. However, in healthy transitions, previous expectations are gradually modified and replaced with new expectations that are realistic for the new situation. In unhealthy transitions, the older adult and family maintain unrealistic expectations and anticipate a future that probably cannot happen.

3. Another characteristic of healthy transitions is the restructuring of life routines. Routines serve to order daily life and provide predictability, manageability, and even pleasure (Cartwright, Archbold, Stewart, & Limandri, 1994). In healthy transitions, routines are restructured in a way that is congruent with the new situation and allows the person to regain a sense that his or her life is predictable, manageable, and pleasurable (Daley, 1993). In unhealthy transitions, such restructuring does not take place. Instead, the older adult attempts to cling to former routines even though they no longer work in the new situation. If the person's abilities and the environment that sustained daily routines are no longer present, an unhealthy transition may lead to no routine at all. In such instances, daily life may become unpredictable, disordered, or empty, particularly for individuals who have a history of orderliness in their lives.

4. Healthy transitions are characterized further by developing new knowledge and skills (Brown, 1995; Edwardson, 1988). Specific needs for knowledge and skills are identified, and opportunities for their development are sought (Davis & Grant, 1994). Over time, the older adult's knowledge and skills closely fit the demands of the new situation. In unhealthy transitions, new knowledge and skills are avoided. Elderly persons and families try to manage the new situation with knowledge and skills that may have been sufficient in the past, but are no longer useful in the present situation. Opportunities for developing knowledge and skills are not taken, resulting in a gap between the demands of the situation and the knowledge and skills available to meet those demands.

5. Although transitions involve endings and disruptions, not everything in the life of the elderly client and his or her family changes. There are continuities, even as change occurs (Burgener, Shimer, & Murrell, 1992; Cartwright et al., 1994). Healthy transitions are characterized by maintaining whatever continuity is possible in identity, relationships, and environment. Continuity facilitates coping with the changes brought about by the transition and fosters the elderly person's ability to integrate the transition experience into his or her life as a whole. In unhealthy transitions, there is discont'nuity and disruption where it does not need to occur. There is lack of awareness of the possibilities for continuity, and change that could be avoided happens anyway. In such instances, transitions become more pervasive than they need to be and older adults sustain losses that could have been prevented.

6. The transitions experienced by elderly persons often are associated with losses, but it is possible that gains occur as well. One of the gains that may be experienced during a transition is the opportunity for new choices (Adlersberg & Thorne, 1990; Happ, Williams, Strumpf, & Burger, 1996). In healthy transitions, the elderly person is open to exploring new choices. He or she engages in seeking and creating new opportunities. Through the exercise of choice, the older adult actively shapes the transition process. Unhealthy transitions are characterized by limiting choices. Older adults themselves may limit the choices available, or choices may be limited by others in the environment (Nick, 1992). The process of limiting choices forecloses possibilities before they are explored. Choices that could be made are passed by, and the elderly person and family are passive with respect to determining the direction of the transition.

7. Finally, healthy transitions are characterized by finding opportunities for personal growth (Langner, 1995; McDougall, 1995; Young, 1990). New levels of self-awareness, new dimensions of identity and relationships, and

new abilities can emerge during transitions. In healthy transitions, such opportunities for growth are embraced in a way that makes personal development and self-actualization possible. In unhealthy transitions, opportunities for growth are rejected. The developmental process is stalled or thwarted in a way that precludes the unfolding and emerging of self.

Process Indicators

As noted previously, process indicators are measurable indices of how a transition is proceeding. Many such process indicators can be used for assessment during a transition. In this chapter, we have identified five for consideration (see Figure 1.1). We present them to exemplify an approach to evaluating the transition process and to stimulate others to identify additional indicators.

1. The elderly person's symptom experience is the first process indicator we consider. During a transition, the older person may experience new symptoms or exacerbation of previously existing symptoms (Ferrell & Schneider, 1988; Kozak, Campbell, & Hughes, 1996). Symptoms should be managed as much as possible so that the elderly person can attend to the transition process itself. If the beginning of the transition is marked by an increase in symptoms, there should be a measurable decline in their frequency and severity over the course of the transition. Although some physical and behavioral symptoms may be inevitable, they should be controlled as much as current symptom management strategies allow. The presence of symptoms that could be controlled suggests that the transition process is proceeding in an unhealthy direction. Patterns of symptoms and the management strategies used by the client should be noted carefully because they provide insight into how the transition is going.

2. Functional status is the next process indicator we propose. For the elderly person, changes in functional status may occur during a transition (Glass & Maddox, 1992; King et al., 1994). However, when a healthy transition process is taking place, the highest possible level of physical and cognitive functioning is achieved over the course of the transition. The elderly person's self-care ability, independence, and mobility are enhanced to the furthest extent possible. A suboptimal level of functioning suggests an unhealthy transition process.

3. Another process indicator is the elderly person's sense of connectedness to a meaningful interpersonal network (Daley, 1993; Rickelman, Gallman, & Parra, 1994; Windriver, 1993). Although disruption in rela-

tionships may occur during a transition, there will be evidence of a regained sense of connectedness when the transition process is proceeding in a healthy direction. If the transition involved loss of one or more relationships, new or transformed relationships should be forged during the transition process to provide a stable source of connectedness by the completion of the transition process. Feelings of disconnectedness or isolation indicate unhealthy transition processes.

4. Another process indicator is a sense of empowerment (Jones & Meleis, 1993; Nyström & Segesten, 1994). The elderly person's sense of autonomy, self-determination, and personal agency may be threatened during the disruption brought about by the transition. However, a new sense of empowerment is found when the transition process is healthy. The older adult regains some control over his or her life. He or she is able to make decisions and put them into effect. For older adults with severe cognitive or physical limitations, there is an appropriate transfer of empowerment to a family member or significant other. Inappropriate disempowerment is indicative of an unhealthy transition process. Disempowerment may be manifested in loss of control, inability to make and carry out decisions, and inappropriate assumption of control by persons in the older adult's environment.

5. The final process indicator we propose is a sense of integrity (Erikson, Erikson, & Kivnick, 1986; Finfgeld, 1995; Mercer, Nichols, & Doyle, 1988). A sense of integrity includes a sense of wholeness and coherence. Personal growth and new insights about self are evidence of a healthy transition. There also is the sense that the transition fits into one's life story in a meaningful way. A loss of integrity indicates an unhealthy transition process. Loss of integrity may be manifested in a sense of fragmentation or meaninglessness in one's life course.

NURSING THERAPEUTICS

The goals of nursing therapeutics from a transition perspective are to facilitate healthy transition processes, to decrease unhealthy transitions, and to support positive process indicators (Meleis & Trangenstein, 1994). Many nursing therapeutics could be used to facilitate transitions. We have selected five for discussion here that we believe have particular relevance for elderly clients (see Figure 1.1). These therapeutics take into account needs specific to this stage of the life cycle, such as the needs for life review and for integration into new living environments. They also take into account challenges often experienced by elderly persons, such as memory loss and changes in mobility.

Nursing Assessment

Nursing assessment is the basis for all nursing therapeutics. The use of a transition perspective suggests several principles for assessment. First, the nature of transitions as dynamic, ongoing processes suggests that nursing assessment must be continuous (McCracken, 1994; Moneyham & Scott, 1995). As the transition evolves, the nurse needs to address changes and developments in the client's situation. Because it is not possible to predict the course of a transition at its outset, assessment must be ongoing. A linear sequence of nursing actions beginning with assessment and moving in turn through planning, implementation, and evaluation is not congruent with a transition perspective. Rather, assessment must span the whole period of transition so that nursing care can evolve along with the movement of the transition process. Such ongoing assessment requires particular vigilance on the nurse's part plus creation of a health care context that supports frequent contact between the nurse and client.

Continuous assessment by the nurse takes into account patterns of transition. Knowing that multiple transitions often occur for elderly persons leads to the anticipation of simultaneous and sequential transitions. For example, knowing that the death of the spouse of a frail elderly person may mean that the elderly person must move from his or her home shapes the nurse's assessment of resources and options for the future. Knowing that a transition for an older adult often has a ripple effect through the family means that a thorough family assessment should be included in the assessment process.

Although assessment is a continuous process for the nurse practicing within a transition perspective, we suggest assessment of the process indicators identified previously at critical points during the transition. The use of process indicators provides the nurse with a way of tracking client progress and provides for early detection of difficulties at critical points in the transition.

The use of formal assessment instruments aids the nurse in making these periodic evaluations of the transition process. They provide an objective measure of the client's situation, allowing the nurse to identify deviations from population norms as well as deviations from the client's own norm. In Table 1.1, we provide examples of tools that could be used to

TABLE 1.1 Tools for Measuring Process Indicators

Symptom Experience
State/Trait Anxiety Inventory (Spielberger, 1983)
Geriatric Depression Scale (Yesavage & Brink, 1983)
Mini-Mental State Questionnaire (Folstein, Folstein, & McHugh, 1975)
McGill Pain Questionnaire (Melzack, 1975)

Functional Status
Index of Activities of Daily Living (Katz, Ford, Moskowitz, Jackson, &
    Jaffe, 1963)
Multidimensional Functional Assessment (Duke University, 1978)

Connectedness
Mutuality Scale (Archbold, Stewart, Greenlick, & Harvath, 1992)
Adult Attachment Scale (Lipson-Parra, 1989)

Empowerment
Desired Control Scale (Reid & Ziegler, 1981)

Integrity
Fulfillment of Meaning Scale (Burbank, 1992)

measure process indicators. The use of process indicators is relevant with family members as well as with elderly persons. The timing and frequency of their use should be determined by the nature of the transition and the extent of the changes it precipitates.

Reminiscence

Reminiscence (Burnside, 1990; Burnside & Haight, 1992) is a nursing therapeutic that facilitates integration of the transition into the life course. Transitions must be viewed within the context of the elderly individual's whole life. Although they involve disruption and change, placing transitions within the context of the life course facilitates the processes of exploring meaning and discovering areas in which continuity with the past is still possible. The articulation of life themes through reminiscing supports the process of growth and development of identity. Reminiscence also can assist the older adult in reinterpreting the meanings of life situations, achieving resolution of ongoing issues, and transcending old pains. Thus reminiscence supports the process of new beginnings as the older adult proceeds through the transition.

Reminiscence is derived from "debriefing," an approach to therapy used with victims of disasters and with individuals who have encountered other crisis situations. Debriefing provides an opportunity to recount the difficult experience and to relive the reactions and emotions that were encountered. Reminiscence is like debriefing in that it provides an opportunity to reflect on important life experiences and to integrate the past into the present. For the person in transition, reminiscence provides an important bridge between the past and present as he or she ends one situation or stage in life and embarks on another.

For older adults with memory loss, the process of reminiscence must be tailored to individual needs. The memories that an older adult has depends on the type and extent of memory loss. Using reminiscence for older adults with memory loss may require innovative strategies (McDougall, 1994; Rentz, 1995). For example, finding a person who serves as a reservoir of memories for an elderly person with memory loss may facilitate reminiscing. The use of prompts, such as photographs or music (Cartwright et al., 1994) also may serve to stimulate memories.

Role Supplementation

Role supplementation is a nursing therapeutic that facilitates the process of developing new knowledge and skills. It is a nursing therapeutic that has been used for parental caregivers (Brackley, 1992), for new parents (Gaffney, 1992; Meleis & Swendsen, 1978; Swendsen, Meleis, & Jones, 1978), for Alzheimer's patients (Kelley & Lakin, 1987), for cardiac rehabilitation (Dracup et al., 1984), and it has much potential for use with elderly persons. Role supplementation provides the support needed to revise continuously skills and capabilities as demands evolve in the new situation. It is defined as the process of bringing into awareness the behaviors, sentiments, sensations, and goals involved in a given role (Meleis, 1975), and it is particularly useful for persons taking on a new role or experiencing a transition in a long-standing role. In the process of role supplementation, information and experiences are conveyed to the role incumbent and his or her significant others so that the role transition can be made smoothly. It includes heightening awareness of one's own role and another's and the dynamics of their interrelationships (Meleis, 1975).

Role supplementation has several components. One is role clarification or the identification of all aspects of a role. For example, role clarification may include a discussion of what is involved in being a nursing home resident. For a family member, it may be the identification of behaviors and feelings associated with the caregiving role. Another component of role supplementation is the process of role taking. Role taking is the empathetic ability to understand the position and point of view of another and to understand how one's role may affect other persons.

Several strategies are used in role supplementation. One is role modeling or the opportunity to observe someone in the role that is being taken on. Another is role rehearsal, the process of mentally or physically enacting the new role that the person is moving toward. Although there are multiple ways of enacting a given role, there are some aspects of roles that tend to be stable and consistent across individuals. For example, although there are some common features of nursing home roles, how they are enacted by a given individual is a dynamic and creative process. Providing clients and their significant others with opportunities to enact and rehearse both the common and creative features of a role leads to greater comfort with the role. Another strategy that facilitates transition for elderly persons and their families is the mobilization of a reference group that is responsive to the various situational and long-term needs of older adults. Reference groups may be for mobility and exercise, for eating, for recreation, and for dealing with chronic illness.

Creation of a Healthy Environment

Another nursing therapeutic for older persons in transition is creation of a healthy environment. We define "environment" broadly to include the older person's physical, social, political, and cultural surroundings. During a transition, the environment itself or the elderly person's interaction with a familiar environment may change. For example, in relocation or migration it is the environment itself that changes. It is the older person's interaction with the environment that changes when a decrease in mobility or cognition limits the ability to function in a familiar environment.

There are many facets to creating a healthy environment. One is to structure the environment so that it provides safety and security (McCracken, 1994; Taft, Delaney, Seman, & Stansell, 1993). Another is to facilitate access to what the elderly person needs and uses to accomplish daily routines (Daly & Berman, 1993). Honoring cultural traditions is another way of creating a healthy environment (Jones, 1995). Finally, freeing the environment of obstacles to dignity and personal integrity fosters a healthy environment (Magee et al., 1993). The use of a transition perspective means that the goal of nursing is the creation of an environment that is dynamic and flexible enough to change in synchrony with the elderly person's evolving needs. It also means that the nurse maintains ongoing involvement with the older adult and family as they continuously modify, restructure, and reinvent the environment to meet the needs of the older family member.

Mobilization of Resources

Older adults in transition face new situations and demands for which previously developed resources may no longer be adequate. Therefore, mobilization of resources is an important aspect of nursing practice within a transition perspective. Enhancement of both personal and environmental resources appropriate to the individual's needs is necessary.

Resources include personal, family, and community resources. Specific resources in each category may be stable or changing, ongoing or newly developed. For example, personal resources may change during a transition, necessitating the mobilization of new personal resources. Similarly, the older adult may have long-standing family resources, but may need additional resources to meet the challenges of a transition. The community resources available to older adults differ according to geographic location and political policies, thus necessitating the ongoing mobilization of new community resources. In short, to mobilize resources, the nurse needs to consider not only the availability of resources, but whether or not they are stable or changing. Also, the nurse must consider whether existing resources are adequate or if new resources must be developed.

Mobilizing personal inner resources is one step toward facilitating healthy transitions in older adults. Scholars variously refer to personal resources as adaptability (Jones, 1991), coherence (Antonovsky, 1987), and hardiness (Kobasa, 1979). Magnani (1990) identified "hardiness" as antecedent to successful aging and recommended that nurses help older adults remain independent and optimize normal healthy aging through three strategies: helping to strengthen the older adult's self-concept, helping the older adult to see his or her life events in perspective, and encouraging appropriate forms of activity.

Another personal resource is wellness (Alford & Futrell, 1992; U.S. Department of Health and Human Services [USDHHS] & American Association for Retired Persons [AARP], 1991; Walker, 1992). A healthy lifestyle should be promoted during a transition. The nurse can encourage regular exercise, a nutritious diet, control of alcohol intake, and abstinence from smoking. Regular primary health care services also are important during a transition.

A strong immune system is another resource that influences the transition process. Exposure to new environmental threats challenges the ability of the immune system to protect the body successfully and maintain physiological integrity. Therefore, promoting activities that strengthen the immune system is one way of mobilizing personal resources. Recent research has demonstrated a variety of behaviors that increase immuno-competence, including laughter (Cousins, 1989), exercise (Nash, 1994), and a positive spirit (Kinion & Kolcaba, 1992). Regular immunizations against influenza and other infectious diseases provide extra immune protection. For some frail elderly persons, a compromised immune system may call for use of antibiotics to prevent as well as to treat infections.

Energy is another personal resource that facilitates smooth transitions. Energy is essential for developing new skills, for pursuing new opportunities for growth, and for maintaining functional status. The mobilization of energy needs to be a deliberate strategy if the older adult is to remain independent and empowered. Proper diet and regular exercise are key factors in energy mobilization. However, energy is holistic; thus psychological, social, and spiritual factors also are significant in its mobilization. These factors influence the older person's motivation to engage actively in life and to seek new opportunities for growth. In the Jones and Meleis (1993) Health Empowerment Model, mobilization of resources is an integral part of promoting energy for health and healthy transitions (see Figure 1.2).

Family resources also may need to be mobilized to assist an aging client in transition. Family resources can be described in terms of structural, economic, and cultural factors. The availability of family members to assist and support an aging person is a primary resource. However, it is possible that even in cultures where caring for aging family members is highly valued, the availability of family caregivers may be limited. In today's global society, family caregivers may be thousands of miles away from the person needing care. Furthermore, whole families may be in transition at the same time, as is the case with immigration. In such instances, the demands on each member are high. Thus consideration of the needs of the whole family is necessary.

Community resources outside of the family may be needed to supplement what the family is able to provide. Some cultural groups tend to do more direct caregiving and to use community services less than others. For example, it has been shown that Blacks and Latinos enter nursing homes at lower rates than do Euro Americans and rely on informal, family-based

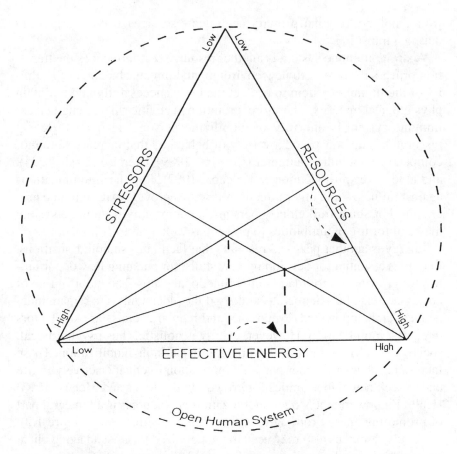

Figure 1.2 Mobilization of resources in the Jones and Meleis Health Empowerment Model (Jones & Meleis, 1993).

support systems to a greater degree than Euro Americans (Angel, Angel, & Himes, 1992). This means that Black and Latino families caring for elderly family members may need more assistance in mobilizing and accessing community resources to support caregiving at home.

Throughout their lives, individuals participate as members of many different communities. Church and community service organizations are examples. In late adulthood, continued contact with members of these communities contributes to a sense of connectedness. The respect, common history, and affirmation that come with membership in these groups contribute to meaning, life satisfaction, and self-esteem.

CASE STUDY

We demonstrate the use of a transition framework in practice by describing a case study. Mr. Adams is a 76-year-old widower whose wife died 1 month following the diagnosis of leukemia. With her illness and death, Mr. Adams entered a period of transition that lasted for over a year. This transition involved his daughter, Gloria White, as well as Mr. Adams. Mrs. White is a middle-aged woman who lives in another country with her husband and teenage children. Prior to her mother's death, Mrs. White visited her parents about once a year. Because of her family responsibilities and the expense of international travel, most of the communication between the Adamses and their daughter had been by telephone.

Mr. Adams had a long history of transient ischemic attacks that occasionally were accompanied by loss of consciousness. These episodes were followed by mental confusion and difficulty with activities of daily living. Prior to her death, Mrs. Adams had provided the assistance that he needed at these times.

After Mrs. Adams' death, family and friends encouraged Mr. Adams to move into a retirement center for increased assistance and social contact. However, he strongly resisted such a move. Throughout his home were pictures, paintings, furniture, and other items that represented significant memories, not only of his wife, but of his own parents and childhood. On the property was a small workshop that housed an elaborate electric train, his lifelong hobby. In the garden were flowers and flowering shrubs that he and his wife had carefully chosen. Mr. Adams became angry and agitated when people encouraged him to move away from this familiar and meaningful environment.

Mr. Adams' health problems, compounded by his grief, emotional distress, and geographical distance from his daughter, worried his next door neighbor. She contacted a gerontological clinical nurse specialist who worked with a local parish nursing program and asked for her advice. With Mr. Adams' permission, the nurse made a home visit and began providing nursing care using a transition perspective. Her initial assessment revealed the physical and emotional symptoms he was experiencing as well as his difficulties with activities of daily living. He felt isolated and alone. He also felt as if his autonomy and rights were being taken away and that he was going to be forced to leave his home. The initial nursing assessment included calls to Mrs. White and a complete assessment of her family responsibilities and resources. The nurse learned that Mrs. White was in the process of getting a divorce and thus was going through a simultaneous transition.

After the initial assessment, the nurse began to assist Mr. Adams with mobilizing community resources to enable him to remain in his home. Obvious needs included assistance with activities of daily living, socialization, and supervision to prevent harm. Assessment of resources also included identifying his own strengths as well as what was necessary to supplement those strengths to continue living independently. Arrangements were made for home care attendants to assist with activities of daily living, domestic chores, grocery shopping, and transportation. Meals on Wheels were arranged, medications were organized for easy administration, and an electronic personal alert system for use in an emergency was set up.

The nurse also helped Mrs. White negotiate the transition in her relationship with her father by assisting her to take on the caregiving role from a distance in the context of multiple family responsibilities and limited financial resources. Areas in which she could provide assistance and support to her father were identified. Also identified were realistic caregiving expectations for her. During this time, Mrs. White was a resource to her father and at the same time was a family member needing support for her own transitions.

Because she realized that major transitions such as loss of one's spouse often are followed by further transitions, the nurse maintained ongoing assessment with Mr. Adams and Mrs. White. For about 6 months, the initial arrangements provided the support Mr. Adams needed and he continued to live at home. Then Mr. Adams' physical health began to decline. His episodes of transient ischemia increased, and he had several falls that caused injuries. It became clear that he could not continue to live alone, and Mrs. White came to help him make decisions and arrangements for a new living situation. He decided to enter a group living center where he could have his own two bedroom duplex, but also would have all the assistance he needed.

In preparation for the move, extensive time was allowed for Mr. Adams to reminisce about the life he had enjoyed in his home. Possessions with special meaning were selected for relocation with him to the new environment. Role supplementation prepared him for his new role in the retirement center. Because the move was another major transition, arrangements were made for his daughter to be present to provide added support during this time.

The move to the assisted living center was difficult for Mr. Adams. He missed his home a great deal and initially had difficulty identifying the new environment as home. For a while his health problems continued with frequent fluctuations in his functional abilities and mental status. However, as the months passed his health stabilized. His emotional well-being increased, and his cognitive status improved. He was able to engage in more self-care and began to participate in activities with other residents. Four months after his relocation, Mr. Adams felt at home in the retirement center. He had made friends there and found that he still had an acceptable degree of autonomy. Also, he had found meaning in assisting a blind resident who needed a companion to accompany him on outings. Mr. Adams expressed to his daughter and friends that the move had turned out to be the right decision after all.

IMPLICATIONS FOR PRACTICE AND KNOWLEDGE DEVELOPMENT

The framework that we have proposed extends our previous work with the concept of transition (Chick & Meleis, 1986; Meleis, 1986; Meleis & Trangenstein, 1994; Schumacher & Meleis, 1994) by identifying specific transition processes, by suggesting indicators of client progress through transitions, and by identifying nursing therapeutics with particular relevance for older clients in transition. We have related transition processes to health by identifying processes that lead to well-being and those that lead to increasing vulnerability. This work is based on the premise that the mission of nursing is to facilitate healthy transitions and to prevent the risks to health that can arise during transitions (Meleis & Trangenstein).

How can this framework be used in clinical practice?

1. It has implications for nursing assessment in that it identifies transition processes with enough specificity to guide observation and interview. The identification of healthy and unhealthy transition processes and indicators provides the nurse with greater ability to assess the direction of the transition and to identify clients at risk.

2. The nursing therapeutics included in the framework can be used to assist clients in many types of transition.

3. The framework can be used to advocate for an approach to practice that values continuity, family centeredness, and wellness.

These nursing values are threatened by a health care climate in which cost cutting is leading to significant constraints on practice. This transition framework provides a way to articulate the complexity of transitions and the resulting need for nursing care that is holistic and continuous.

The framework also can be used to guide knowledge development through theory and research. Questions it suggests include: (1) How do different patterns of transition influence transition processes and process indicators? (2) What are the critical periods in the various patterns? (3) What are the relationships between patterns of transition and patterns of nursing intervention? To address these questions, preliminary work will be needed, including further description of transition patterns, processes, and process indicators; identification or development of additional tools for measurement; and continued specification and refinement of nursing therapeutics.

We conclude by emphasizing the importance of a transition perspective in gerontological nursing. Older adults experience multiple transitions related to their health and well-being. These transitions are not short-lived events. Rather, they are complex processes that evolve over a period of time and usually involve a number of individuals. To make nursing practice congruent with the experiences of older adults, the nurse must view their needs from a perspective that takes into account the complexity and temporal characteristics of the experience. We argue that a transition perspective provides the gerontological nurse with a powerful means of understanding and responding to the needs of older adults. We challenge gerontological nurses to use, refine, and extend the framework we have described.

REFERENCES

Ade-Ridder, L., & Kaplan, L. (1993). Marriage, spousal caregiving, and a husband's move to a nursing home: A changing role for the wife? *Journal of Gerontological Nursing, 19* (10), 13–23.

Adlersberg, M., & Thorne, S. (1990). Emerging from the chrysalis: Older widows in transition. *Journal of Gerontological Nursing, 16*(1), 4–8.

Alford, D. M., & Futrell, M. (1992). AAN working paper: Wellness and health promotion of the elderly. *Nursing Outlook, 5,* 221–226.

Angel, R. J., Angel, J. L., & Himes, C. L. (1992). Minority group status, health transitions, and community living arrangements among the elderly. *Research on Aging, 14,* 496–521.

Antonovsky, A. (1987). *Unraveling the mystery of health.* San Francisco: Jossey-Bass.

Archbold, P. G., Stewart, B. J., Greenlick, M. R., & Harvath, T. A. (1992). The clinical assessment of mutuality and preparedness in family caregivers to frail older people. In S. G. Funk, E. M. Tornquist, M. T. Champagne, & R. A. Wiese (Eds.), *Key aspects of elder care: Managing falls, incontinence, and cognitive impairment* (pp. 328–339). New York: Springer.

Brackley, M. H. (1992). A role supplementation group pilot study: A nursing therapy for potential parental caregivers. *Clinical Nurse Specialist, 6*, 14–19.

Bridges, W. (1980). *Transitions*. Reading, MA: Addison-Wesley.

Brown, D. S. (1995). Hospital discharge preparation for homeward bound elderly. *Clinical Nursing Research, 4*, 181–194.

Bull, M. J. (1992). Managing the transition from hospital to home. *Qualitative Health Research, 2*, 27–41.

Bull, M., Jervis, L. L., & Her, M. (1995). Hospitalized elders: The difficulties families encounter. *Journal of Gerontological Nursing, 21*(6), 19–23.

Bull, M. J., Maruyama, G., & Luo, D. (1995). Testing a model for posthospital transition of family caregivers for elderly persons. *Nursing Research, 44*, 132–138.

Burbank, P. (1992). Assessing the meaning of life among older adult clients. *Journal of Gerontological Nursing, 18*(9), 19–28.

Burgener, S. C., Shimer, R., & Murrell, L. (1992). Expressions of individuality in cognitively impaired elders: Need for individual assessment and care. *Journal of Gerontological Nursing, 19*(4), 13–22.

Burnside, I. (1990). Reminiscence: An independent nursing intervention for the elderly. *Issues in Mental Health Nursing, 11*, 33–48.

Burnside, I., & Haight, B. K. (1992). Reminiscence and life review: Analyzing each concept. *Journal of Advanced Nursing, 17*, 855–862.

Cartwright, J. C., Archbold, P. G., Stewart, B. J., & Limandri, B. (1994). Enrichment processes in family caregiving to frail elders. *Advances in Nursing Science, 17*(1), 31–43.

Chick, N., & Meleis, A. I. (1986). Transitions: A nursing concern. In P. L. Chinn (Ed.), *Nursing research methodology: Issues and implementation* (pp. 237–257). Rockville, MD: Aspen.

Conn, V. S., Taylor, S. G., & Messina, C. J. (1995). Older adults and their caregivers: The transition to medication assistance. *Journal of Gerontological Nursing, 21*(5), 33–38.

Cousins, N. (1989). *Head first: The biology of hope*. New York: E. P. Dutton.

Daley, O. E. (1993). Women's strategies for living in a nursing home. *Journal of Gerontological Nursing, 19*(9), 5–9.

Daly, M. P., & Berman, B. M. (1993). Rehabilitation in the elderly patient with arthritis. *Clinics in Geriatric Medicine, 9*, 783–801.

Davis, L. L., & Grant, J. S. (1994). Constructing the reality of recovery: Family home care management strategies. *Advances in Nursing Science, 17*(2), 66–76.

Dewar, A. L., & Morse, J. M. (1995). Unbearable incidents: Failure to endure the experience of illness. *Journal of Advanced Nursing, 22*, 957–964.

Dracup, K., Meleis, A. I., Clark, S., Clyburn, A., Shields, L., & Staley, M. (1984). Group counseling in cardiac rehabilitation: Effect on patient compliance. *Patient Education and Counseling, 6*, 169–177.

Duke University Center for the Study of Aging and Human Development. (1978). *Multidimensional functional assessment: The OARS methodology*. Durham, NC: Duke University.

Edwardson, S. R. (1988). Outcomes of coronary care in the acute care setting. *Research in Nursing & Health, 11*, 215–222.

Erikson, E. H., Erikson, J. M., & Kivnick, H. Q. (1986). *Vital involvement in old age*. New York: W. W. Norton.

Ferrell, B. R., & Schneider, C. (1988). Experience and management of cancer pain at home. *Cancer Nursing, 11*, 84–90.

Finfgeld, D. L. (1995). Becoming and being courageous in the chronically ill elderly. *Issues in Mental Health Nursing, 16*, 1–11.

Folstein, M. F., Folstein, S. E., & McHugh, P. R. (1975). Mini-Mental State: A practical method for grading the cognitive state of patients for the clinician. *Journal of Psychiatric Research, 12*, 189–198.

Gaffney, K. F. (1992). Nursing practice model for maternal role sufficiency. *Advances in Nursing Science, 15*(2), 76–84.

Glass, T. A., & Maddox, G. L. (1992). The quality and quantity of social support: Stroke recovery as psycho-social transition. *Social Science and Medicine, 34*, 1249–1261.

Happ, M. B., Williams, C. C., Strumpf, N. E., & Burger, S. G. (1996). Individualized care for frail elders: Theory and practice. *Journal of Gerontological Nursing, 22*(3), 6–14.

Johnson, M. A., Morton, M. K., & Knox, S. M. (1992). The transition to a nursing home: Meeting the family's needs. *Geriatric Nursing, 13*, 299–302.

Jones, P. S. (1991). Adaptability: A personal resource for health. *Scholarly Inquiry for Nursing Practice, 5*, 95–112.

Jones, P. S. (1995). Paying respect: Care of elderly parents by Chinese and Filipino American women. *Health Care for Women International, 16*, 385–398.

Jones, P. S., & Meleis, A. I. (1993). Health is empowerment. *Advances in Nursing Science, 15*(3), 1–14.

Katz, S., Ford, A. B., Moskowitz, R. W., Jackson, B. W., & Jaffe, M. (1963). Studies of illness in the aged. The index of ADL, a standardized measure of biological and psychosocial function. *Journal of the American Medical Association, 185*, 914–919.

Kelley, L. S., & Lakin, J. A. (1987). Role supplementation as a nursing intervention for Alzheimer's disease: A case study. *Public Health Nursing, 5*, 146–152.

King, K. B., Porter, L. A., & Rowe, M. A. (1994). Functional, social, and emotional outcomes in women and men in the first year following coronary artery bypass surgery. *Journal of Women's Health, 3,* 347–354.

Kinion, E. S., & Kolcaba, K. Y. (1992). Plato's model of the psyche: A holistic model for nursing interventions. *Journal of Holistic Nursing, 10,* 218–230.

Kobasa, S. C. (1979). Stressful life events, personality, and health: An inquiry into hardiness. *Journal of Personality and Social Psychology, 37,* 1–11.

Kozak, C. J., Campbell, C., & Hughes, A. M. (1996). The use of functional consequences theory in acutely confused hospitalized elderly. *Journal of Gerontological Nursing, 22*(1), 27–36.

Langner, S. R. (1995). Finding meaning in caring for elderly relatives: Loss and personal growth. *Holistic Nursing Practice, 9*(3), 75–84.

Lipson-Parra, H. (1989). Development and validation of the Adult Attachment Scale: Assessing attachment in elderly adults. *Issues in Mental Health Nursing, 11,* 79–92.

Magee, R., Hyatt, E. C., Hardin, S. B., Stratmann, D., Vinson, M. H., & Owen, M. (1993). Institutional policy: Use of restraints in extended care and nursing homes. *Journal of Gerontological Nursing, 19*(4), 31–39.

Magnani, L. E. (1990). Hardiness, self-perceived health, and activity among independently functioning older adults. *Scholarly Inquiry for Nursing Practice: An International Journal, 4,* 171–185.

McCracken, A. L. (1994). Special care units: Meeting the needs of cognitively impaired persons. *Journal of Gerontological Nursing, 20*(4), 41–46.

McDougall, G. (1994). Mental health and cognition. In P. Ebersole & P. Hess (Eds.), *Toward healthy aging: Human needs and nursing response* (4th ed., pp. 612–657). St. Louis: Mosby.

McDougall, G. J. (1995). Existential psychotherapy with older adults. *Journal of the American Psychiatric Nurses Association, 1,* 16–21.

Meleis, A. I. (1975). Role insufficiency and role supplementation: A conceptual framework. *Nursing Research, 24,* 264–271.

Meleis, A. I. (1986). Theory development and domain concepts. In P. Moccia (Ed.), *New approaches to theory development* (pp. 3–21). New York: National League for Nursing.

Meleis, A. I., & Swendsen, L. A. (1978). Role supplementation: An empirical test of a nursing intervention. *Nursing Research, 27,* 11–18.

Meleis, A. I., & Trangenstein, P. A. (1994). Facilitating transitions: Redefinition of the nursing mission. *Nursing Outlook, 42,* 255–259.

Melzack, R. (1975). The McGill Pain Questionnaire: Major properties and scoring. *Pain, 1,* 277–299.

Mercer, R. T., Nichols, E. G., & Doyle, G. C. (1988). Transitions over the life cycle: A comparison of mothers and nonmothers. *Nursing Research, 37,* 144–150.

Michels, N. (1988). The transition from hospital to home: An exploratory study. *Home Health Care Services Quarterly, 9*(1), 29–44.

Moneyham, L., & Scott, C. B. (1995). Anticipatory coping in the elderly. *Journal of Gerontological Nursing, 21*(7), 23–28.

Nash, M. S. (1994). Exercise and immunology. *Medicine & Science in Sports & Exercise, 26,* 125–127.

Nick, S. (1992). Long-term care. Choices for geriatric residents. *Journal of Gerontological Nursing, 18*(7), 11–28.

Nyström, A. E. M., & Segesten, K. M. (1994). On sources of powerlessness in nursing home life. *Journal of Advanced Nursing, 19,* 124–133.

Reid, D. W., & Ziegler, M. (1981). The desired control measure and adjustment among the elderly. In H. M. Lefcourt (Ed.), *Research with the locus of control construct: Vol. 1. Assessment methods* (pp. 127–157). New York: Academic Press.

Rentz, C. A. (1995). Reminiscence: A supportive intervention for the person with Alzheimer's disease. *Journal of Psychosocial Nursing and Mental Health Services, 33*(11), 15–20.

Rickelman, B. L., Gallman, L., & Parra, H. (1994). Attachment and quality of life in older, community-residing men. *Nursing Research, 43,* 68–72.

Schumacher, K. L., & Meleis, A. I. (1994). Transitions: A central concept in nursing. *Image: Journal of Nursing Scholarship, 26,* 119–127.

Spielberger, C. D. (1983). *Manual for the State-Trait Inventory (STAI) Form Y.* Palo Alto, CA: Consulting Psychologists Press.

Stewart, B. J., Archbold, P. G., Harvath, T. A., & Nkongho, N. O. (1993). Role acquisition in family caregivers for older people who have been discharged from the hospital. In S. G. Funk, E. M. Tornquist, M. T. Champagne, & R. A. Wiese (Eds.), *Key aspects of caring for the chronically ill: Hospital and home* (pp. 219–231). New York: Springer.

Swendsen, L. A., Meleis, A. I., & Jones, D. (1978). Role supplementation for new parents: A role mastery plan. *American Journal of Maternal Child Nursing, 3,* 84–91.

Taft, L. B., Delaney, K., Seman, D., & Stansell, J. (1993). Creating a therapeutic milieu in dementia care. *Journal of Gerontological Nursing, 19*(10), 30–39.

U.S. Department of Health and Human Services, & American Association for Retired Persons. (1991). *Healthy older adults 2000.* Washington, DC: AARP Health Advocacy Services.

Walker, S. N. (1992). Wellness for elders. *Holistic Nursing Practice, 7*(1), 38–45.

Wilson, S., & Billones, H. (1994). The Filipino elder: Implications for nursing practice. *Journal of Gerontological Nursing, 20*(8), 31–36.

Windriver, W. (1993). Social isolation: Unit-based activities for impaired elders. *Journal of Gerontological Nursing, 19*(3), 15–21.

Yesavage, J. A., & Brink, T. L. (1983). Development and validation of a geriatric depression screening scale. A preliminary report. *Journal of Psychiatric Research, 17,* 37–49.

Young, H. M. (1990). The transition of relocation to a nursing home. *Holistic Nursing Practice, 4*(3), 74–83.

CHAPTER 2

Retirement: Health Issues, Perspectives, and Policy Considerations

Lorraine T. Dorfman and Carla Gene Rapp

R etirement is one of the major role transitions of later life in modern industrialized societies. As a result of lengthening life expectancy, retirement also occupies a steadily increasing portion of the life course and characterizes growing numbers of older people, thus commanding more attention from professionals and the public. Retirement can affect virtually all aspects of an individual's life, not least among them health, which has a complex and not fully understood relationship to retirement. Many important questions concerning health and retirement deserve further exploration, including the effect of health on the retirement decision, the effects of retirement on health, the relationship between health and adjustment to retirement, the financing of health care in retirement, and gender, socioeconomic, and ethnic group variations. Considerable confusion and misconceptions exist about some of these questions.

This chapter provides a synthesis of recent research on health and retirement. We first examine the effect of health on the decision to retire. We then review research on the effects of retirement on physical and mental health, and the relationship between health and retirement adjustment. We go on to look at several health care issues in retirement, including health insurance coverage and health care in residential retirement settings, and conclude with implications for nursing practice, research, and policy. We provide a context for these issues by turning first to some recent trends in retirement.

DEFINITIONAL ISSUES AND RECENT TRENDS

Retirement can be seen in a number of different ways—as an event, a process that occurs over time, a new social role that one plays, or a phase of life (Atchley, 1976). It can be defined by various objective criteria, or subjectively by the individual who sees himself or herself as retired. These different definitions obviously make a difference in who is considered "retired." Although multiple criteria often are used in assessing retirement status, the ones most often utilized are (a) level of activity in the labor market and (b) receipt of some sort of pension. These two criteria are commonly operationalized as (a) separation from a job or occupation that was the person's life work, (b) change from full-time employment to either no employment or to a different job requiring fewer hours, or no more than a specified number of hours per week or number of weeks or months per year, and (c) acceptance of Social Security or other public or private pension benefit (Atchley, 1976; Ekerdt & DeViney, 1990; Holden, 1989).

Retirement was not institutionalized in the United States until late in the 19th century when industrialization enabled older individuals to withdraw from the workforce and still receive an income based on their prior work contribution (Atchley, 1976, 1997). Graebner (1980), in tracing the evolution of retirement, noted that retirement really emerged in the 20th century as a way to restructure the workforce and was a result of the movement toward efficiency in the workplace. Retirement was democratic in the sense that it was universal and egalitarian, and it was used as a way to try to deal with the unemployment of younger persons (Graebner). By the 1960s, as private and public pensions increased and Social Security benefits were broadened, retirement became much more embedded in the social fabric.

A long-term trend toward earlier retirement, particularly for men, has been evident since the middle of this century. Nearly half (49.9%) of men age 65 were in the labor force in 1970, compared to only about three tenths (29.9%) of men age 65 in 1993. Labor force participation of men age 62, the earliest age of Social Security receipt, showed a similar pattern of decline; indeed, by 1993, just over half of men (51.5%) were still in the labor force by age 62 (Atchley, 1997). Some indication of a leveling off in the rate of early labor force withdrawal for men occurred during the 1980s; in fact, there was a small increase in labor force participation among men in the older age groups. Between 1985 and 1995, labor force participation among men ages 65–69 increased from 24.5% to 27.0%, and it also increased somewhat among men in their 70s (Hurd, 1996). Whether this increase signals a long-term change in patterns of labor force participation among older men remains to be seen.

The labor force participation of older women shows a different pattern from that of men, as it has remained relatively stable over time. Labor force participation of women age 65 declined only slightly between 1970 and 1993, from 22.1% to 20.6%, and among women age 62, it merely declined from 36.1% in 1970 to 35.4% in 1993 (Atchley, 1997). These gender differences may reflect in part the overall trend of increased labor force participation of women (Hurd, 1996).

As we approach the end of the 20th century, the transition from work to retirement is becoming increasingly complex. More people are retiring gradually rather than abruptly, returning to work after they retire, and experiencing second and even third retirements. Bridge jobs to retirement may occur for a period of time after leaving one's career job; these jobs are often part-time and at a lower occupational and pay level than career jobs (Atchley, 1997). Older people may reduce their time commitment to work by working fewer weeks or months per year or by working fewer days or hours per week. Henretta (1997) notes that these trends are resulting in "blurred" rather than "crisp" retirements. Blurred retirements may raise additional questions about how to ensure an orderly flow of people into and out of the workforce, and they may confound issues of evaluation of job performance in later life.

THE IMPACT OF HEALTH ON THE DECISION TO RETIRE

Overview

Poor health is clearly one of the major reasons for involuntary and often premature retirement. Atchley (1997) points out that about one third of the population ages 55–64 has a disability severe enough to either limit employment or cause withdrawal from the labor force. Some of these individuals will retire because of their health, while others will draw disability payments until they become eligible for retirement benefits. Several researchers, using national datasets such as the Social Security Administration New Beneficiary Survey, the National Longitudinal Surveys of Labor Market Experience, and the new Health and Retirement Survey (Burkhauser, Couch, & Phillips, 1996; Ozawa & Law, 1992; Parnes & Less, 1985; Sherman, 1985) report that poor health is the most common reason given for involuntary retirement, and they estimate that health-induced withdrawal from the labor force ranges from 25% to above 35%. Many of these unhealthy individuals also have lower monthly earnings, lower receipt of pensions, and fewer assets than do individuals who do not retire because of poor health (Ozawa & Law). They are therefore more likely to suffer lower levels of economic well-being in retirement, including poverty, than are their healthy counterparts (Burkhauser et al.).

One of the problems that plagues researchers in assessing the magnitude of retirement due to ill health is that health may sometimes be given as a convenient excuse for retiring when the reason is actually something else. For example, some retirees may prefer to say that they retired because of their health rather than say they were forced out of their jobs (Parnes & Less, 1985). Poor health may therefore provide an acceptable rationale for retiring for the individual whose job is eliminated through organizational downsizing or who is forced to take early retirement (Juster & Suzman, 1995). At least one study, however, found that persons who retired because of poor health were indeed impaired over a wide range of functional, affective, and memory behaviors (Colsher, Dorfman, & Wallace, 1988).

Several investigators have examined the relationship between specific health conditions and the work-retirement decision. Wray (1996) reported increased odds of being retired for older persons who have circulatory and heart conditions or diabetes, whereas Sarfas (1993) found that back injury was the most common cause of retirement because of health. In a population-based survey of rural elderly persons, Colsher et al. (1988) found that a lifetime history of several life-threatening health conditions increased the probability of health-related retirement, most notably myocardial infarction, stroke, and diabetes for men, and cancer, diabetes, and hip fracture for women. Several minor health conditions also increased the probability of health-related retirement among women, but not among men, in that study. Taken together, these studies suggest that cardiovascular and cerebrovascular problems, diabetes, and musculoskeletal conditions are leading causes of health-induced retirement.

Racial, Ethnic, and Gender Differences

A number of racial and ethnic minorities including African Americans, Puerto Ricans, and Mexican Americans experience poorer health and more disability than do nonminorities, which contributes to their disadvantage in both work and retirement (Bound, Schoenbaum, & Waidmann, 1996; Gibson & Burns, 1991; Hayward & Liu, 1992; Wray, 1996). The poorer work status and disadvantaged retirement status of those minorities result from many factors, among them overrepresentation in low status or physically demanding jobs, less access to high quality health services, and inability to afford good medical care (Cowan, 1978; Gibson & Burns). African-American men and women, for example, are much more likely to report that they are physically unable to work than are Whites (Bound et al.), leading often to an "unretired-retired" status for older African Americans (Gibson, 1993; Gibson & Burns). Nonparticipation in the labor force linked to physical disability rather than to retirement may result in a disabled, rather than a retired, identity (Gibson & Burns). Zsembek and Singer (1990) note some similarities in the situation of older Mexican Americans to that of African-American older adults. These findings suggest that older minorities may not fit conventional definitions of "retirement." In fact, Hayward and Liu conclude that retirement is more of a White than an African-American experience, whereas disability is more of an African-American than a White experience.

With regard to gender differences about health and the decision to retire, older men are more likely to report life-threatening health conditions such as cardiovascular disease and cancer than are women (Herzog, 1989). It is not unreasonable to expect that older men with those serious health conditions will retire. Data from two large surveys indicate that health limitations and poorer self-rated health are predictors of retirement among men, but not among women (George, Fillenbaum, & Palmore, 1984).

THE EFFECTS OF RETIREMENT ON HEALTH

Myths and misconceptions abound concerning the effects of retirement on health. In particular, a widely held belief purports that retiring is harmful to one's health and may even hasten death, despite rather consistent evidence to the contrary. Ekerdt (1987), in a seminal article titled "Why the Notion Persists that Retirement Harms Health," offers several reasons:

(1) anecdotal evidence of persons whose health failed just after retiring (although those persons usually had preexisting health conditions); (2) attribution of causality to a major life event that causes change; (3) the cultural celebration of work in our society; (4) certain theoretical frameworks such as activity theory and stressful life events theory suggesting that lack of full social participation and stressful life events increase the likelihood of illness; and (5) misinterpretation of research findings. We turn now to the empirical evidence of the effects of retirement on health status.

Physical Health

Virtually all studies agree that retirement has little, if any, negative effect on physical health (e.g., Ekerdt, Baden, Bossé, & Dibbs, 1983; Ekerdt & Bossé, 1982; Ekerdt, Sparrow, Glynn, & Bossé, 1984; Herzog, House, & Morgan, 1991; Hibbard, 1995). In longitudinal studies of men who participated in the Veterans Administration Normative Aging Study, Ekerdt and his colleagues found no significant differences in changes in physical health over 3 to 4 years between men who retired and their same-age peers who remained employed (Ekerdt, Baden, Bossé et al., 1983). Objective measures of health in that study included physical exams, blood and urine analyses, chest X rays, and ECGs. Likewise, Ekerdt and Bossé observed that self-reports of change in health status did not differ significantly between men who retired and men who remained employed. Few men (2%) in the Normative Aging Study said that retiring had a "bad" effect on their health, whereas nearly half (48%) said that retirement had a "good" effect on their health (the remaining 50% claimed no effect) (Ekerdt & Bossé). Additionally, pre- to postretirement change in level of somatic complaints did not differ significantly between those retired men and their age peers who continued to work (Ekerdt, Bossé, & Goldie, 1983), nor were there clinically significant changes in blood pressure or cholesterol level between the two groups (Ekerdt et al., 1984).

Studies of older women also show few, if any, negative effects of retirement on health status. Follow-ups of Swedish women 5 months after their retirement revealed that blood pressure, musculoskeletal symptoms, and calls to physicians had declined from measurements taken 6 months prior to retirement. Additionally, 22% of the women reported health improvement after retirement, whereas only 9% reported health deterioration (Ostberg & Samuelsson, 1994). Using data from the National Center for Health Statistics' Longitudinal Study on Aging, Hibbard (1995) found that women age 70 and older who had been in the workforce and who had more recent employment (age 45+) reported better health, had fewer Activities of Daily Living (ADL) and Instrumental Activities of Daily Living (IADL) limitations, and fewer functional limitations than did women who had not been in the workforce or who had less recent employment. Although it is possible that the working women experienced better health all along, this study provides no evidence to suggest that employed women suffer ill-health effects after they retire.

Misconceptions also abound about the positive effects of retirement on health. It is not unreasonable to expect some benefits resulting from retirement because of reduced role strain and demands that were formerly associated with employment. The evidence, however, is that retirement does not seem to improve health for most people, with the possible exception of those who retire for health-related reasons (Ekerdt, Bossé, & LoCastro, 1983; Ogunbameru, 1993). Thirty-eight percent of the men in the Veterans Administration Normative Retirement Study claimed that retirement had improved their health; however, retrospective claims of improved health were not supported by longitudinal data (Ekerdt, Bossé, & LoCastro, 1983). Interestingly, men who claimed that retirement had improved their health were also those who had been employed in more physically demanding and mentally and emotionally stressful jobs. The elimination of strain associated with those jobs may help explain the men's perception of improved health after retirement.

Mental Health

Most people adjust well to retirement and do not experience persistent feelings of stress, dissatisfaction, anxiety, or depression associated with retirement. Approximately one third of retirees, however, do experience adjustment problems, and a few never adapt to retirement (Atchley, 1997; Bossé, Aldwin, Levinson, & Workman-Daniels, 1991). Mental health professionals need to direct particular attention to the group of retirees that cannot adapt especially if adjustment problems appear to persist over time, because of the effects of poor adjustment on physical, psychological, and social functioning.

One way to try to understand the effect of retirement on mental health is to conceptualize retirement as an evolving experience that is likely to vary considerably over time. Atchley (1976) provided a model of phases of retirement that may help us understand retirement as a process. First is a preretirement phase, both remote and near, with the near stage marked by some negative feelings, worries, and fears about retirement. This is followed by a honeymoon phase, during which time retirees may experience a sense of euphoria and try to do too much with their newfound free time. A period of disenchantment may then set in, where there may be some letdown and depression. The next two phases are reorientation, for those retirees who have become upset or depressed, and stability, where life regains a more reasonable balance and tempo. The last phase of retirement, according to Atchley's model, is a termination phase characterized by illness and, perhaps, disability. It is important to point out that the timing of these phases of retirement is seen as variable, and that not all retirees can be expected to experience all of the phases in sequence, thus providing a degree of flexibility in the retirement experience (Atchley, 1976).

Several studies have provided empirical support for the phases of Atchley's model, particularly its early phases. Retirees appear to experience a positive effect of retirement somewhere during the 1st year after retiring, as evidenced by feelings of enhanced well-being, increased interpersonal and life satisfaction, and reduction of anxiety (Ekerdt, Bossé, & Levkoff, 1985; Gall, Evans, & Howard, 1997; Richardson & Kilty, 1995), thus suggesting a honeymoon phase shortly after the retirement event occurs. Feelings of enhanced well-being, including less depression than prior to retirement, have also been reported during the 2nd year of retirement (Midanik, Soghikian, Ransom, & Tekawa, 1995; Reitzes, Mutran, & Fernandez, 1996). Other research, in contrast, has found that life satisfaction and overall psychological health may decline between the 1st and 2nd year of retirement, indicating that feelings of letdown and disenchantment may begin to surface once the early sense of euphoria of fades (Ekerdt et al., 1985). Longitudinal research on retirees over a longer period suggests that a period of reorientation and stability may follow a period of disenchantment, with retirees showing a high overall level of life satisfaction even after 6 or 7 years of retirement, although not as high a level of satisfaction as during early retirement (Gall et al.).

One of the factors that may affect mental health in retirement is one's attitude toward retirement. Daly and Futrell (1989) studied a number of health outcomes in retirement in relation to preretirement attitudes and found that a positive attitude toward retirement was the strongest predictor of emotional health in retirement for both men and women. Interestingly, that study also found that a positive attitude toward retirement was the strongest predictor of physical health for men and women.

Several problematical behaviors, such as alcoholism, abuse of other substances, and even suicide have been thought to be linked with retirement because of job-related loss of status and self-esteem and retirees not having enough activity to fill each day. One could argue, alternatively, that the probability of such problem behaviors is lessened after retiring because of the elimination of work-related stress. Few studies focus on these issues. Comparing men who retired with men who remained employed in a 2-year follow-up from preretirement, Ekerdt, DeLabry, Glynn, and Davis (1989) concluded that retirement did not cause a big shift in the average amount of alcohol consumption or drinking behaviors. However, retired men appeared to show more variability in drinking than did men who continued to work; some retirees showed lighter drinking, while others showed heavier drinking and more problems with drinking than did their employed counterparts. The relationship between alcohol use and retirement thus appears to be complex and warrants further investigation. With respect to suicide, it is difficult to establish a causal link between retirement and suicide because many other factors such as bereavement, poor health, depression, alcohol abuse, and living arrangements can affect whether a person is likely to attempt suicide (Templer & Cappelletty, 1986). Evidence from one study, however, indicates that involuntary retirement is associated with an increased likelihood of contemplating suicide (Peretti & Wilson, 1978). What this suggests is that older people who are forced into a major life change such as retirement may become unhappy enough to at least consider suicide.

HEALTH AND THE ADJUSTMENT TO RETIREMENT

Health is identified as a major determinant of retirement adjustment in virtually all retirement studies. Other factors associated with positive adjustment to retirement (as measured by retirement satisfaction, overall life satisfaction, happiness, and morale) include adequate finances (Beck, 1982; Calasanti, 1988; Dorfman, Kohout, & Heckert, 1985; Gall et al., 1997; Palmore, Burchett, Fillenbaum, George, & Wallman, 1985), positive attitude toward retirement (Daly & Futrell, 1989; Streib & Schneider, 1971; Thompson, Streib, & Kosa, 1960), voluntary rather than forced retirement (Gall et al.; Kimmel, Price, & Walker, 1978; Peretti & Wilson,

1975), higher occupational status (Richardson & Kilty, 1991; Streib & Schneider), and continued social participation (Dorfman et al., 1985; Dorfman & Rubenstein, 1993; Hooker & Ventis, 1984; Lemon, Bengston, & Peterson, 1972; Palmore et al.).

Good health gives older persons the opportunity to engage in a wide variety of retirement activities, such as volunteer or community service, hobbies, social activities, and leisure time pursuits that they may have long planned for. Health limitations, on the other hand, particularly those associated with serious health conditions, can result in a spoiled retirement. Individuals who retire because of poor health often say that retirement is worse than they expected, that they are dissatisfied with retirement, or that there is nothing they like about retirement (Crowley, 1985; McGoldrick & Cooper, 1994). Good health, then, can be seen as a retirement resource that, if not available, impedes enjoyment of retirement.

Although the evidence is consistent regarding the effects of overall health status on retirement adjustment, much less is known about the effects of specific health conditions on retirement adjustment. Dorfman (1995), in the first study of its kind, examined the effects of specific health conditions on quality of life in retirement, as measured by dimensions of retirement satisfaction. Pulmonary disease was a predictor of dissatisfaction with health for retired men and women. Additionally, heart attack and stroke were predictors of dissatisfaction with health and activities for men, whereas arthritis was a predictor of dissatisfaction with health for women. These findings suggest that programs and services may need to be targeted to retirees with particular health conditions, and also to the specific needs of retired men and women.

THE FINANCING OF HEALTH CARE IN RETIREMENT

Health care costs must be taken into account when making the decision to retire, as most Americans who have health insurance receive this insurance as a benefit of working. Some employers provide health insurance as a postretirement benefit, while other retirees choose to purchase an individual plan. Medicare covers approximately 96% of Americans age 65 or older, and Medicaid may be available for a portion of retirees as well (Snider, 1994). Generally, older adults spend more on their health care than do younger adults. The possibility of needing long-term care increases with age, thus making financing of health care a serious concern for most retirees.

Currently, the majority of American retirees obtain both income (Social Security) and health care benefits (Medicare) from the federal government; however, the financial viability of these programs is uncertain. The 1997 Annual Report of the Boards of Trustees of the Social Security and Medicare trust funds recounts the actuarial status of these funds. The Medicare trust fund is projected to be unable to pay benefits on time and in full starting between mid-2000 and early 2001. Social Security fund exhaustion is expected to occur in 2029; however, the fund's expenditures will exceed current tax income beginning in 2012 (Anonymous, 1997).

This information is not new; in fact, starting in 1993, the Boards of Trustees have notified Congress yearly about the potential exhaustion of these funds (Anonymous, 1996). Unless action is taken rapidly, these funds will be depleted and government support for older adults will be drastically changed in the 21st century. Although attention should be paid to the predicted Social Security fund exhaustion, the rapidly approaching exhaustion of the Medicare fund is an emergency that must be addressed promptly. Recent changes have been made to both the Social Security and Medicare programs as a result of the 1997 Balanced Budget Act. Although the actual actuarial effect on the trust funds is not yet clear, certainly, an increase in solvency will result.

Pensions and Social Security Income

Two common sources of income for retirees are Social Security and employer-sponsored pensions. Currently, the most common "normal" retirement age is 65, since this is the earliest age one can receive full Social Security benefits. Most other pension plans use age 65 as their retirement age as well. In 1983, the Social Security Act was amended in an effort to alleviate the projected shortfall in that fund; this amendment will result in the "normal" retirement gradually rising to age 67 by 2027 (Chen, 1994). Private pensions are expected to follow suit as well. One concern about increasing normal retirement age is whether older people will remain in the labor market. Questions exist about elderly workers' ability to work, as well as the willingness of employers to hire older workers (Chen).

Some retirees choose to retire earlier than age 65, and Social Security does provide this option. People may choose to retire at age 62 and receive 80% of the benefits that they would have received at age 65. The 1983 legislation will decrease the proportion of income available to early retirees from 80% to 70% by 2027 (Chen, 1994).

Historically, firms offered early retirement to lower current labor costs by replacing older workers with younger workers who might receive lower salaries (Clark, Ghent, & Headen, 1994; Hirshorn, Tetrick, & Sinclair, 1996; Russell, 1996). In the absence of retiree health insurance, the high cost of individual health insurance for persons ages 50 to 64 may discourage older workers from retiring during this time frame. Many workers wait until they are Medicare eligible before retiring. Hirshorn et al. surveyed companies and found that 35.2% provided health care benefits, 71.7% provided pensions, and only 32.4% provided both pensions and health care benefits to their retirees.

Medicare

Medicare provides hospital insurance (Part A) and supplementary medical insurance (Part B) for most retirees. Deductibles and copayments are required; these usually rise each year. Prescription drugs, eyeglasses, hearing aids, dentures, and routine health checkups are not included in Medicare coverage, and there is very little coverage of long-term care (Atchley, 1997; Chen, 1994; Herzog, 1989).

Despite recent congressional action, the Medicare trust fund continues to have financing problems. More and more, politicians and policy makers are becoming aware of this impending disaster, and some attempts are being made to avert the shortfall. One of the most common questions asked is, "How did this happen?" Bagby (1997) points out that when Medicare was founded, the ratio of contributors to beneficiaries was 8:1; now the ratio has dropped to 4:1, and it is predicted to continue to drop. The cost of Medicare is high for a variety of reasons: (a) the cost of administration and bureaucracy has increased; (b) "defensive medicine" has increased health care costs; (c) new technologies have added to health care costs; and most important (d) the number of elderly persons is increasing rapidly (Bagby; Lubitz, Beebe, & Baker, 1995).

Managed care has been suggested as a possible solution to health care financing problems in general, as well as for the Medicare system. Butler, Sherman, Rhinehart, Klein, and Rother (1996) discuss the advantages and disadvantages of managed care, specifically health maintenance organizations (HMO) for the Medicare population. Identified advantages include (a) emphasis on prevention, (b) increased flexibility in care delivery, and (c) fewer restrictions and wider coverage (e.g., dental care provided and prescriptions filled) than Medicare fee-for-service. Disadvantages include (a) limited access to and choice of health care and/or providers, and (b) a potential for professional conflict of interest (Butler et al.).

One suggestion is that Medicare could become part of, or be restructured to resemble, the Federal Employees Health Benefits Program (FEHBP) (Butler & Moffit, 1995; McArdle, 1995). This plan, which was created by Congress in 1959, is actually more of a purchasing pool than an insurance plan. In this plan, the amount that the FEHBP pays to a member is pre-set, and he or she can choose how to spend that money (Butler & Moffit). McArdle suggests that although the FEHBP is not a perfect plan, it success can provide options when proposing health care reform.

Medicaid

Medicaid is the federal health insurance program for the poor, no matter what their age. For some retirees, Medicaid funds are used to help pay for Medicare premiums, deductibles, and copayments (Merrell, Colby, & Hogan, 1997); other retirees access Medicaid after entering a long-term care (LTC) facility (Butler, 1996; Hudson, 1995; Wiener, 1996).

Hudson (1995) discusses the ethical dilemma facing policy makers concerning how Medicaid moneys should be spent. Because Medicaid is the only federal program that pays for LTC, this program is being used by 6 of every 10 nursing home residents (Hudson). Although elderly persons make up only one quarter of Medicaid beneficiaries, they account for two thirds of the expenditures, with 33% of the money being spent on LTC (Wiener, 1996).

Because of the high use of Medicaid funds by elderly persons, this area often is suggested as a target in spending cuts. Butler (1996) cautions that changes to both Medicaid and Medicare may inequitably affect older women because women have increased longevity as well as an increased likelihood of poverty and institutionalization compared to men. Wiener (1996) examined methods to decrease Medicaid spending on LTC, focusing on ways to change eligibility for these funds. He concluded that the current system of gaining Medicaid eligibility for LTC is "actually pretty economical" (p. 810).

Private Health Insurance

The majority of older adults have health care coverage through Medicare; however, approximately 80% of older adults have some sort of private health insurance as well, whether as a retiree benefit from a past employer or through the purchase of an individual plan (Lillard, Rogowski, & Kington, 1997; Morrisey, 1993). Chulis, Eppig, Hogan, Waldo, and Arnett (1993) found that only 11% of Medicare beneficiaries did not have additional insurance coverage (employer-sponsored retiree coverage or individually purchased coverage) or Medicaid. Unfortunately, research shows a declining trend in employer-sponsored retiree health insurance coverage (Clark et al., 1994; Lillard et al.).

In 1990, Congress enacted legislation that standardized coverage offered in supplemental health insurance ("medigap" policies) designed for older adults (Fox, Rice, & Alecxih, 1995). Although the standardization reduces consumer choice, it also should facilitate comparison shopping. Morrisey (1993) found that approximately 50% of retirees have some form of medigap coverage. In general, private health insurance coverage is most likely among persons who are enrolled in Medicare, more educated, younger, female, White, residing in the Midwest or Northeast, in good physical health, and with higher incomes (Morrisey; Wilcox-Gok & Rubin, 1994).

Only a small minority of retirees currently have LTC insurance, which can cover both nursing home care and in-home care. Enrollment in LTC policies is increasing, however, as this insurance continues to improve. Cohen, Kumar, and Wallack (1994) suggest voluntary purchase of LTC insurance by individuals as a way to help cut Medicaid costs. These authors found that in the presence of LTC insurance, only 8% to 10% of all policyholders would receive Medicaid.

RETIREMENT RELOCATION

Persons 65 and older choose to live in a variety of locations. Although stereotypically, older Americans relocate on retirement, Walsh (1992) points out that older adults are actually less likely than any other age group to change place of residence. Therefore, it can be expected that the majority of older adults' living arrangements will remain the same as when they were middle-aged.

A variety of factors impact on the older adult's decision to relocate upon retirement, including desired location, desired services, desire to be around age peers, the retiree's physical and mental abilities, safety issues, transportation, community support, and availability of caregivers (Rapp,

1996; Silverstein & Zablotsky, 1996). Retirees may decide to move to share a home, most often with a family member or friend, move into a mobile home, or "live" in a recreational vehicle. Some older adults choose to live in retirement communities. These communities can be single buildings, neighborhoods of private homes, or preplanned housing developments (which often include single- and multifamily dwellings as well as apartments). Naturally occurring retirement communities are found in areas where large numbers of retirees live. Planned retirement communities are usually age segregated and aggressively marketed. Continuing care retirement communities (CCRCs) generally offer independent living, assisted living, and nursing home care.

Silverstein and Zablotsky (1996) investigated the likelihood of moving to a retirement community. They found that retirees were increasingly likely to move to a retirement community as a disability advanced to moderate levels, but became less likely when a disability was severe. Institutionalization became more likely as a disability worsened. Elderly persons who lived alone or whose children did not live nearby were likely to move to a retirement community. The authors concluded that relocation to a retirement community is triggered not only by desired social and amenity opportunities, but also by the need for assistive services as a result of physical frailty (Silverstein & Zablotsky).

HEALTH CARE IN RETIREMENT
RESIDENTIAL SETTINGS

This discussion will focus on services provided in continuing care retirement communities (CCRCs) because these retirement settings offer the fullest variety of health care services. Although "home care" is not always offered in CCRCs, brief mention will be made of these services because many retirees will receive in-home care.

Home Care

Recently, the distinctions between home care and residentially based care have begun to blur. Kane (1995) reports that some care providers are offering services, including personal assistance, to people who are not homebound, or who live in apartment complexes or assisted living facilities. In fact, entrepreneurs are suggesting the creation of group residential settings where consumers with severe disabilities can receive personal care and nursing in their own apartments. This type of arrangement is attractive to elderly persons who wish to retain more control over their lives than is currently available in most LTC institutions. State regulations may be a potential limiting factor in the development of such residentially oriented LTC programs (Kane).

Continuing Care Retirement Communities

CCRCs offer housing, health care, social support, and other amenities specifically targeted to older adults. Health services generally include personal and nursing home care, but they also may include primary and preventive care (Gupta & Galanos, 1996; Sloan, Shayne, & Conover, 1995). Three different types of CCRCs exist:

1. Type A CCRCs (extensive facilities) require a very large entrance fee, and residents pay the same monthly fee no matter what level of care is utilized. This type of facility guarantees coverage of LTC needs.

2. Type B CCRCs (modified facilities) have a smaller entrance and monthly fee, and agree to provide a limited amount of health and nursing home care for the monthly fee, with other services available at additional cost.

3. Type C CCRCs (fee-for-service facilities) provide housing and amenities for a minimal entrance and monthly fee, plus easy access to further health and nursing home services, but these are all paid for on a fee-for-service basis (Brower, 1994; Petit, 1994; Sloan et al.).

The reasons retirees move to a CCRC are similar to the reasons any retiree relocates; however, Gupta and Galanos (1996) found that health was the most frequently reported reason for relocation to a CCRC. Other reasons cited were climate and proximity to family, convenience of amenities provided, and provision of long-term security for a spouse. The authors concluded that retirees saw relocation as a way to ensure their continuing independence (Gupta & Galanos).

Major concerns for many older adults when considering joining a CCRC is the large financial investment required and the possibility of bankruptcy. Conover and Sloan (1995) found that CCRC bankruptcy rates are very low (annual rate of .3%), with failure rates equivalent to that of health insurance in general. CCRCs have been suggested as a model for use in revising LTC delivery because they offer a full continuum of services and can substitute less expensive supportive care for institutional care (Brower, 1994; Sloan et al., 1995). Research shows that having personal care services in the independent living setting or the assisted living setting in any of the CCRC types reduces nursing home use. Specifically, extensive CCRCs were more likely to provide supportive services that allowed the resident to stay in the lower cost setting (independent instead of assisted, and assisted instead of a nursing home) (Sloan et al.).

IMPLICATIONS FOR NURSING

The most important role for a nurse in regard to retirement is that of information provider and educator. Nurses also act as consultant, adviser, and advocate for older persons as they make their decision to retire and then adapt to this new role. Nurses should be alert to signs of adjustment problems, such as depression, which can occur shortly after the retirement event or may develop later in retirement. They should be sure to address the widely held misapprehension that retiring is harmful to one's health. Retirees should know that retirement appears to have little effect on physical health, either negatively or positively, although the way a person perceives his or her health may change. Thus one is not too surprised to find that a positive attitude toward retirement is a predictor of postretirement mental and physical health. Positive attitudes may be fostered through anticipatory guidance. Much of retirement planning should begin long before the actual age of retirement; thus nongerontologic nurses can assist in this process.

Similarly, negative behaviors (substance abuse and suicide) seem more likely in people who retire involuntarily. Nurses should be sure to assess for indicators of these problems when dealing with persons who did not have much control over their retirement. On the basis of what is known about dissatisfaction with retirement, programs and services could be targeted to retirees with particular health conditions (pulmonary disease for both genders; heart attack and stroke for men; arthritis for women) who have been found to be most dissatisfied with their health.

Nurses should remember that health-induced retirement is more likely in persons with cardiovascular and cerebrovascular problems, diabetes, and musculoskeletal conditions; therefore, care plans should address this possibility. Older minority clients are less likely to fit the conventional definitions of retirement, and also are more likely to be poor and in ill health. Women are especially vulnerable to impoverishment during retirement, on the basis of their lifetime income history, increased longevity, and increased risk of institutionalization.

The financial status of many of our retired clients is already fairly well determined; however, nurses can assist in a more global way by being active in the political arena to try to positively affect policy related to federal programs for elderly persons (Social Security and Medicare). Additionally, nurses should discuss investment in private pensions and purchase of individual health insurance, especially long-term-care coverage, with their clients. The reality is that the federal programs are in serious danger and Americans must change their mind-set about government assistance. No longer are Social Security and Medicare given expectations: retired Americans may be increasingly responsible for their own income and health care costs. Although the outcome of the impending changes is not known, nurses can help prepare older adults to deal with the transition by providing advice and referral.

New models of care are being developed to attempt to meet the health care needs of the rapidly increasing number of older adults. Older retired adults are becoming more vocal about their desire to remain in their homes and communities as they age, and our models are beginning to change from institutional to assistive and supportive ones. In the future, the models of assistive living and life care (as seen in CCRCs) will be areas that nurses must know. Clients will expect nurses to provide counseling to older persons on the benefits and pitfalls of these more independent living and health care models, as well as expect nurses to influence health care policy.

Nurses have a history of being creative problem solvers, of assessing situations and integrating data, and communicating with others in an attempt to provide optimal care for their clients. In the future, nurses will need to use all of their skills to help clients prepare for, make the transition into, and then adjust to retirement. Hard decisions are going to have to be made about Social Security and Medicare, and nurses must be vocal in this policy-making process, both as patient advocates and to ensure that nursing services will be provided to retirees.

CONCLUSIONS AND FUTURE DIRECTIONS

Several conclusions can be drawn from the research on health and retirement reviewed in this chapter. It is clear that health is a major factor in the decision to retire, and that it contributes to an earlier than anticipated retirement for some older people. Retirement in itself, however, has little, if any, adverse effects on health, despite widely held beliefs to the contrary. Some retirees even believe that retiring improves their health. Most people adjust well to retirement, which is facilitated by good health. A minority of retirees, on the other hand, exhibit adjustment problems such as depression, feelings of dissatisfaction, and behavioral problems, thus offering a challenge to mental health professionals. Other challenges to professionals who work with retired populations include the provision of appropriate health care in various residential settings, and uncertainties surrounding the financing of such health care.

Significant gaps remain in our knowledge about the relationship between health and retirement. Much of the research in the area is cross-sectional in design or based on short-term longitudinal studies. Both physical and mental health status may change markedly over the course of retirement; therefore, long-term studies that follow retirees over a period of years are needed. Information gained from longitudinal research also is imperative if we are to understand better the transition to retirement. About one third of retirees have some problems in adapting to this life transition (Atchley, 1997; Bossé et al., 1991). It also would be valuable to investigate the mental and physical health status of individuals who retire primarily for health reasons, not just initially, but at various intervals during the retirement years to see how they fare over the course of retirement compared to individuals who retire for other reasons.

Progress has been made in examining gender differences in work and retirement patterns; however, more information is needed on possible cohort differences in the health and retirement experiences of women and men. Although older women typically have had very different employment histories than have older men, cohorts of younger women, including those born in the "baby boom" generation, are more likely to spend a greater proportion of their lives in the workforce, thus more closely resembling the work patterns of men. Likewise, considerably more research is needed that will explore variations in health, employment, and retirement of racial and ethnic minorities, who are expected to comprise a significantly larger percentage of older adults in the next century than they do today. Some research exists on the retirement of African Americans and Mexican Americans, but there is a paucity of information about other minorities, including recent immigrants from Asia and the Pacific Islands.

Research on the effect of retirement housing choice has implications for both policy makers and practitioners. Comparative studies of health care needs along the continuum from independent to completely dependent retirement residential settings can help in the design of appropriate health interventions by nurses and other professionals. Such information is particularly important as retirees age and move into group housing, assisted living facilities, and CCRCs.

A final direction for the future, suggested by our review, is in the area of health promotion, since good health facilitates adjustment to retirement. Health promotion programs for retirees have been observed to improve health risk status and to reduce health care costs (Fries, Bloch, Harrington, Richardson, & Beck, 1993). In designing such health promotion programs, it may be worthwhile to consider programming targeted to the needs of retirees with specific health conditions, such as cardiovascular disease or diabetes (Dorfman, 1995).

More and more older people are living to experience the retirement years. It is very important to conduct research that will contribute to our understanding of retirement and its interrelationship with health. Such research contributes not only to basic knowledge in the area, but can inform policy and practice. Research from nursing as well as other disciplines should be encouraged.

REFERENCES

Anonymous. (1996). Actuarial status of the Social Security and Medicare trust funds. *Social Security Bulletin, 59*(2), 57–63.

Anonymous. (1997). A summary of the 1997 annual report [On-line]. Available: www.ssa.gov.

Atchley, R. C. (1976). *The sociology of retirement.* Cambridge, MA: Schenkman.

Atchley, R. C. (1997). *Social forces and aging* (8th ed.). Belmont, CA: Wadsworth.

Bagby, R. J. (1997). The future of Medicare. *Journal of the Florida Medical Association, 84*, 75–76.

Beck, S. H. (1982). Adjustment to and satisfaction with retirement. *Journal of Gerontology, 37*, 616–624.

Bossé, R., Aldwin, C. M., Levenson, M. R., & Workman-Daniels, K. (1991). How stressful is retirement? Findings from the Normative Aging Study. *Journal of Gerontology: Psychological Sciences, 46*, P9–P14.

Bound, J., Schoenbaum, M., & Waidmann, T. (1996). Race differences in labor force attachment and disability status. *The Gerontologist, 36*, 311–319.

Brower, H. T. (1994). Policy implications for life care environments. *Journal of Gerontological Nursing, 20*, 17–22.

Burkhauser, R. V., Couch, K. A., & Phillips, J. W. (1996). Who takes early Social Security benefits? The economic and health characteristics of early beneficiaries. *The Gerontologist, 36*, 789–799.

Butler, R. N. (1996). On behalf of older women. Another reason to protect Medicare and Medicaid. *New England Journal of Medicine, 334*, 794–796.

Butler, R. N., Sherman, F. T., Rhinehart, E., Klein, S., & Rother, J. C. (1996). Managed care: What to expect as Medicare-HMO enrollment grows. *Geriatrics, 51*(10), 35–42.

Butler, S. M., & Moffit, R. E. (1995). The FEHBP as a model for a new Medicare program. *Health Affairs, 14*(4), 47–61.

Calasanti, T. M. (1988). Participation in a dual economy and adjustment to retirement. *International Journal of Aging and Human Development, 26*, 13–27.

Chen, Y. P. (1994). "Equivalent retirement ages" and their implications for Social Security and Medicare financing. *The Gerontologist, 34*, 731–735.

Chulis, G. S., Eppig, F. P., Hogan, M. O., Waldo, D. R., & Arnett, R. H. D. (1993). Health insurance and the elderly. *Health Affairs, 12*(1), 111–118.

Clark, R. L., Ghent, L. S., & Headen, A. E., Jr. (1994). Retiree health insurance and pension coverage: Variations by firm characteristics. *Journal of Gerontology: Social Sciences, 49*, S53–S61.

Cohen, M. A., Kumar, N., & Wallack, S. S. (1994). Long-term care insurance and Medicaid. *Health Affairs, 13*(4), 127–139.

Colsher, P. L., Dorfman, L. T., & Wallace, R. B. (1988). Specific health conditions and work-retirement status among the elderly. *Journal of Applied Gerontology, 7*, 485–503.

Conover, C. J., & Sloan, F. A. (1995). Bankruptcy risk and state regulation of continuing care retirement communities. *Inquiry, 32*, 444–456.

Cowan, B. (1978). Urban blacks in retirement: Current status, prospects and issues. In E. P. Stanford (Ed.), *Retirement: Concepts and realities of ethnic minority elders* (pp. 75–82). San Diego: San Diego State University, University Center on Aging.

Crowley, J. E. (1985). Longitudinal effects of retirement on men's psychological and physical well-being. In H. S. Parnes (Ed.), *Retirement among American men* (pp. 147–173). Lexington, MA: D. C. Heath.

Daly, E. A., & Futrell, M. (1989). Retirement attitudes and health status of preretired and retired men and women. *Journal of Gerontological Nursing, 15*, 29–32.

Dorfman, L. T. (1995). Health conditions and perceived quality of life in retirement. *Health and Social Work, 20*, 192–199.

Dorfman, L. T., Kohout, F. J., & Heckert, D. A. (1985). Retirement satisfaction in the rural elderly. *Research on Aging, 7*, 577–599.

Dorfman, L. T., & Rubenstein, L. M. (1993). Paid and unpaid activities and retirement satisfaction among rural seniors. *Physical and Occupational Therapy in Geriatrics, 12*, 45–63.

Ekerdt, D. J. (1987). Why the notion persists that retirement harms health. *The Gerontologist, 27*, 454–457.

Ekerdt, D. J., Baden, L., Bossé, R., & Dibbs, E. (1983). The effect of retirement on physical health. *American Journal of Public Health, 73*, 779–783.

Ekerdt, D. J., & Bossé, R. (1982). Change in self-reported health with retirement. *International Journal of Aging and Human Development, 15*, 213–223.

Ekerdt, D. J., Bossé, R., & Goldie, C. (1983). The effect of retirement on somatic complaints. *Journal of Psychosomatic Research, 27*, 61–67.

Ekerdt, D. J., Bossé, R., & Levkoff, S. (1985). An empirical test for phases of retirement: Findings from the Normative Aging Study. *Journal of Gerontology, 40*, 95–101.

Ekerdt, D. J., Bossé, R., & LoCastro, J. S. (1983). Claims that retirement improves health. *Journal of Gerontology, 38*, 231–236.

Ekerdt, D. J., DeLabry, L. O., Glynn, R. J., & Davis, R. W. (1989). Change in drinking behaviors with retirement: Findings from the normative aging study. *Journal of Studies on Alcohol, 50*, 347–353.

Ekerdt, D. J., & DeViney, S. (1990). On defining persons as retired. *Journal of Aging Studies, 4*, 211–229.

Ekerdt, D. J., Sparrow, D., Glynn, R. J., & Bossé, R. (1984). Change in blood pressure and total cholesterol with retirement. *American Journal of Epidemiology, 120*, 64–71.

Fox, P. D., Rice, T., & Alecxih, L. (1995). Medigap regulation: Lessons for health care reform. *Journal of Health Politics, Policy & Law, 20*, 31–48.

Fries, J. F., Bloch, D. A., Harrington, H., Richardson, N., & Beck, R. (1993). Two–year results of a randomized controlled trial of a health promotion program in a retiree population: The Bank of America Study. *The American Journal of Medicine, 94*, 455–462.

Gall, T. L., Evans, D. R., & Howard, J. (1997). The retirement adjustment process: Changes in the well-being of male retirees across time. *Journal of Gerontology: Psychological Sciences, 52B*, P110–P117.

George, L. K., Fillenbaum, G. G., & Palmore, E. (1984). Sex differences in the antecedents and consequences of retirement. *Journal of Gerontology, 39*, 364–371.

Gibson, R. C. (1993). Aging in black America. In J. S. Jackson, L. M. Chatters, & R. J. Taylor (Eds.), *Aging in black America* (pp. 277–297). Newbury Park, CA: Sage.

Gibson, R. C., & Burns, C. J. (1991). The work, retirement, and disability of aging minorities. *Generations, 15*(4), 31–35.

Graebner, W. (1980). *A history of retirement: The meaning and function of an American institution*. New Haven, CT: Yale University Press.

Gupta, N., & Galanos, A. N. (1996). Why healthy elders move to a continuing care retirement community. *North Carolina Medical Journal, 57*, 378–380.

Hayward, M. D., & Liu, M. (1992). Men and women in their retirement years. In

M. Szinovacz, D. J. Ekerdt, & B. H. Vinick (Eds.), *Families and retirement* (pp. 23–50). Newbury Park, CA: Sage.

Henretta, J. C. (1997). Changing perspectives on retirement. *Journal of Gerontology: Social Sciences, 52B*, S1–S3.

Herzog, A. R. (1989). Physical and mental health of older women: Selected research issues and data sources. In A. R. Herzog, K. C. Holden, & M. M. Seltzer (Eds.), *Health and economic status of older women* (pp. 35–91). Amityville, NY: Baywood.

Herzog, A. R., House, J. S., & Morgan, J. N. (1991). Relation of work and retirement to health and well-being in older age. *Psychology and Aging, 6*, 202–211.

Hibbard, J. H. (1995). Women's employment history and their post-retirement health and resources. *Journal of Women and Aging, 7*(3), 43–55.

Hirshorn, B. A., Tetrick, L. E., & Sinclair, R. R. (1996). Understanding the provision of postretirement health care and pension benefits: Which firm characteristics are most explanatory? *The Gerontologist, 36*, 637–648.

Holden, K. C. (1989). Economic status of older women: A summary of selected research issues. In A. R. Herzog, K. C. Holden, & M. M. Seltzer (Eds.), *Health and economic status of older women* (pp. 92–130). Amityville, NY: Baywood.

Hooker, K., & Ventis, D. G. (1984). Work ethic, daily activities, and retirement satisfaction. *Journal of Gerontology, 39*, 478–484.

Hudson, T. (1995). Medicaid: Will the public program neglect the poor to pay for the elderly? *Hospitals & Health Networks, 69*(10), 28–30, 32, 34.

Hurd, M. D. (1996). *Economics of aging interest group newsletter* [Research note]. Washington, DC: Gerontological Society of America.

Juster, F. T., & Suzman, R. (1995). An overview of the health and retirement study. *The Journal of Human Resources, 30* (Suppl. 95), S7–56.

Kane, R. A. (1995). Expanding the home care concept: Blurring distinctions among home care, institutional care, and other long-term-care services. *Milbank Quarterly, 73*, 161–196.

Kimmel, D. C., Price, K. F., & Walker, J. W. (1978). Retirement choice and retirement satisfaction. *Journal of Gerontology, 33*, 573–585.

Lemon, B. W., Bengston, V. L., & Peterson, J. A. (1972). An exploration of the activity theory of aging: Activity types and life satisfaction among in-movers to a retirement community. *Journal of Gerontology, 27*, 511–523.

Lillard, L., Rogowski, J., & Kington, R. (1997). Long-term determinants of patterns of health insurance coverage in the Medicare population. *The Gerontologist, 37*, 314–323.

Lubitz, J., Beebe, J., & Baker, C. (1995). Longevity and Medicare expenditures. *New England Journal of Medicine, 332*, 999–1003.

McArdle, F. B. (1995). Opening up the Federal Employees Health Benefits Program. *Health Affairs, 14*(2), 40–50.

McGoldrick, A. E., & Cooper, C. L. (1994). Health and ageing as factors in the retire-
    ment experience. *European Work and Organizational Psychologist, 4*, 1–20.
Merrell, K., Colby, D. C., & Hogan, C. (1997). Medicare beneficiaries covered by
    Medicaid buy-in agreements. *Health Affairs, 16*(1), 175–184.
Midanik, L. T., Soghikian, K., Ransom, L. J., & Tekawa, I. S. (1995). The effect
    of retirement on mental health and health behaviors: The Kaiser Permanente
    Retirement Study. *Journal of Gerontology: Social Sciences, 50B*, S59–S61.
Morrisey, M. A. (1993). Retiree health benefits. *Annual Review of Public Health,
    14*, 271–92.
Ogunbameru, O. A. (1993). The relationship between health and retirement:
    Evidence from Ondo State, Nigeria. *Journal of Applied Social Sciences, 17*,
    43–56.
Ostberg, H., & Samuelsson, S. M. (1994). Occupational retirement in women due
    to age. *Scandinavian Journal of Social Medicine, 22*, 90–96.
Ozawa, M. N., & Law, S. W. (1992). Reported reasons for retirement: A study of
    recently retired workers. *Journal of Aging and Social Policy, 4*, 35–51.
Palmore, E. B., Burchett, B. M., Fillenbaum, G. G., George, L. K., & Wallman,
    L. M. (1985). *Retirement: Courses and consequences.* New York: Springer.
Parnes, H. S., & Less, L. J. (1985). The volume and pattern of retirements,
    1966–1981. In H. S. Parnes (Ed.), *Retirement among American men* (pp.
    57–77). Lexington, MA: D. C. Heath.
Peretti, P. O., & Wilson, C. (1975). Voluntary and involuntary retirement of aged
    males and their effect on emotional satisfaction, usefulness, self-image, emo-
    tional stability, and interpersonal relationships. *International Journal of Aging
    and Human Development, 6*, 131–138.
Peretti, P. O., & Wilson, C. (1978). Contemplated suicide among voluntary and
    involuntary retirees. *Omega, 9*, 193–201.
Petit, J. M. (1994). Continuing care retirement communities and the role of the
    wellness nurse. *Geriatric Nursing, 15*, 28–31.
Rapp, C. G. (1996). Problems with living arrangements. In A. S. Staab & L. C.
    Hodges (Eds.), *Essentials of gerontological nursing: Adaptation to the prob-
    lems of aging.* Philadelphia: Lippincott.
Reitzes, D. C., Mutran, E. J., & Fernandez, M. E. (1996). Does retirement hurt
    well-being? Factors influencing self-esteem and depression among retirees
    and workers. *The Gerontologist, 36*, 649–656.
Richardson, V. E., & Kilty, K. M. (1991). Gender differences in mental health
    before and after retirement: A longitudinal analysis. *Journal of Women and
    Aging, 7*, 19–35.
Russell, T. E. (1996). Trav'lin' light: Early retirees and the availability of post-
    retirement health benefits. *American Journal of Law & Medicine, 22*,
    537–562.
Sarfas, H. (1993). Ill health retirement in health care workers. *Occupational
    Health: A Journal for Occupational Health Nurses, 45*(3), 101, 103.

Sherman, S. R. (1985). Reported reasons retired workers left their last job: Findings from the New Beneficiary Survey. *Social Security Bulletin, 48*(3), 22–30.

Silverstein, M., & Zablotsky, D. L. (1996). Health and social precursors of later life retirement-community migration. *Journal of Gerontology: Social Sciences, 51*(Suppl.), S150–S156.

Sloan, F. A., Shayne, M. W., & Conover, C. J. (1995). Continuing care retirement communities: Prospects for reducing institutional long-term care. *Journal of Health Politics, Policy & Law, 20*, 75–98.

Snider, S. (1994). Who are the medically uninsured in the United States? *Statistical Bulletin—Metropolitan Insurance Companies, 75*(2), 20–30.

Streib, G., & Schneider, C. (1971). *Retirement in American society.* Ithaca, New York: Cornell University Press.

Templer, D. I., & Cappelletty, G. G. (1986). Suicide in the elderly: Assessment and intervention. *Clinical Gerontologist, 5*, 475–487.

Thompson, W., Streib, G., & Kosa, J. (1960). The effect of retirement on personal adjustment: A panel analysis. *Journal of Gerontology, 14*, 165–169.

Walsh, M. B. (1992). The frail elderly population. In M. M. Burke & M. B. Walsh (Eds.), *Gerontological nursing: Care of the frail elderly* (pp. 1–48). St Louis: Mosby.

Wiener, J. M. (1996). Can Medicaid long-term care expenditures for the elderly be reduced? *The Gerontologist, 36*, 800–811.

Wilcox-Gok, V., & Rubin, J. (1994). Health insurance coverage among the elderly. *Social Science & Medicine, 38*, 1521–1529.

Wray, L. A. (1996). The role of ethnicity in the disability and work experience of preretirement-age Americans. *The Gerontologist, 36*, 287–298.

Zsembek, B. A., & Singer, A. (1990). The problem of defining retirement among minorities: The Mexican-Americans. *The Gerontologist, 30*, 749–757.

CHAPTER 3

Helping Older Adults Adjust to Relocation: Nursing Interventions and Issues

Rebecca A. Johnson

Rapid expansion of the population of older adults in the previous and forthcoming decades is a commonly recognized demographic phenomenon. As larger numbers of older adults attain greater age, with gradually decreasing functional ability, there will be an increased need for appropriate housing options. Statistical predictions indicate that individuals over age 65 have a 43% risk of relocation to a nursing home (Murtaugh, Kemper, & Spillman, 1990). Because of the likelihood that older adults will relocate as they advance in age, and the attendant needs that they have during the process of relocation, this topic is of particular importance to nurses. Additionally, nurses in fulfilling their roles of teachers, advocates and caregivers, may be the health care professionals who are best positioned to assist relocating older adults.

This chapter will articulate the state of knowledge derived from research conducted during the past 20 years about relocation, a transition for older adults, and will discuss interventions to facilitate positive adjustment to this transition. The discussion will center on interventions that have been tested and found to be effective. Additional interventions, the effects of which are as yet empirically unclear in the context of relocation, will also be discussed.

Author Notes: The author wishes to acknowledge the assistance of Norman Shirk, graduate student, Northern Illinois University, for his work in compiling the literature used in this chapter.

RELOCATION AS TRANSITION

Relocation has been defined as the change in environment that takes place when an individual moves from one location to another. It occurs as a process, including changes in the life situation that stimulate the move, the actual physical move, and the adjustment to new surroundings (Remer & Buckwalter, 1990). Older adults may relocate to different communities or within communities. Within or between communities, they may relocate from their own homes to more supportive housing such as apartments, assisted living facilities, retirement communities, or nursing homes. Or they may change locations within supportive housing facilities after having already lived there for a period. Each relocation is a life transition for older adults.

Transitions have been defined as passages or movements from one phase of life, status, condition or place to another (Chick & Meleis, 1986). Three types of transition comprise the model of transition articulated by Chick and Meleis, major concepts of which provide a useful framework for considering relocation. Each transition occurs in a different context and each produces different needs in the person experiencing transition. The three types of transition include developmental, situational, and health-illness transitions. A fourth type of transition, organizational transition, was added to the model at a later date (Schumaker & Meleis, 1994).

Developmental transitions occur as an outgrowth of natural processes associated with maturation throughout the life course, such as retiring or becoming a grandparent. Situational transitions occur as life circumstances change, such as becoming widowed or homeless. Health-illness transitions occur in response to changes in health status or subsequent treatment regimens. Relocation of older adults may be viewed as either a developmental, situational or health-illness transition, or a combination of transition types.

In the transition model, nurses help those experiencing transitions by applying therapeutic nursing interventions. The goal of these interventions is to promote healthy transitions and minimize negative consequences of transitions such as relocation. Interventions are aimed at assessing readiness for the relocation through participation in the decision-making process, preparing for relocation, and supplementing the older adult's ability to adapt to the changes associated with the relocation.

RESEARCH FINDINGS ON
RELOCATION TRANSITIONS

Whatever the settings involved with relocation, this transition may be stressful for older adults because of the extent to which changes occur in the location of their homes necessitating changes in daily routines and support networks. When older adults relocate to more supportive housing, they must learn and live by policies and regulations of the facility. Because relocation is recognized as a stressful life transition, recently the nursing diagnosis of relocation stress syndrome (RSS) was formally identified within nursing (Barnhouse, Brugler, & Harkulich, 1992).

Types of Relocation Transitions

Relocation as a Developmental Transition

Relocation has been perceived as a developmental transition occurring in tandem with maturational processes of individuals and families (Uhlenberg, 1995; Yee & Van Arsdol, 1977). While the first relocation usually occurs shortly after retirement and may be stimulated by the attraction of available amenities at the new location, it often involves long distances (Haas & Serow, 1993; Litwak & Longino, 1987; Speare & Meyer, 1988). This type of relocation occurs in approximately 5% of persons above age 60 who move annually (Litwak & Longino). Older adults commonly relocate to states with high levels of unemployment (Serow, 1987), and from metropolitan areas to nonmetropolitan areas (Clifford, Heaton, & Fuguitt, 1982). Favored locations include Florida, Arizona, Texas, and California (Flynn, Longino, Wiseman, & Biggar, 1985).

Relocation as a Situational Transition

Older adults also may relocate because of changes in their environment or life circumstances, such as loss of a spouse, lack of a kinship network (Freedman, Berkman, Rapp, & Ostfeld, 1994), adult children (Freedman, 1996), or caregiver (Montgomery & Kosloski, 1994), caregiver burden (Cohen, Gold, Shulman, Wortley, McDonald, & Wargon, 1993), financial difficulties, lack of available assistive services (Collins, King, & Kokinakis, 1994), or the goal of improving their living conditions. Or they may be affected by changes in the structure or function of supportive housing facilities where they live, thus requiring relocation (Hallewell, Morris, & Jolley, 1994). For example, in an early study of relocation (Aldrich & Mendkoff, 1963), older nursing home residents ($N = 233$) were transferred from one nursing home to another, to hospitals, to homes of relatives or friends, or to independent community dwellings. The relocation was involuntary because their nursing home was closed.

Relocation as a Health-Illness Transition

Relocation also may occur when chronic diseases, declining functional ability (Colsher & Wallace, 1990; Johnson, Schwiebert, & Alvarado Rosenmann, 1994; Speare, Avery, & Lawton, 1991; Wolinsky, Callahan, Fitzgerald, & Johnson, 1993; Young, Forbes, & Hirdes, 1994), falls (Dunn, Furner, & Miles, 1993), cognitive impairment (Abraham, Currie, Neese, Yi, & Thompson-Heisterman, 1994; Lord, 1994; Osterweil, Martin, & Syndulko, 1995), or psychiatric illness (Goetz & Stebbins, 1994) make it necessary for older adults to seek housing that is nearer to adult children or is more supportive in nature. This transition usually occurs in mid to late old age. Litwak and Longino (1987) identify this relocation using population statistics that show that only 15.5% of older adults moving to Florida are above age 75 compared with 40.6% of those moving north from Florida. A related finding indicated that 11.2% of those moving north from Florida were institutionalized versus 1.2% who moved to Florida from the North.

Outcomes of Relocation Transitions

According to the transition model articulated by Schumacher and Meleis (1994), positive outcomes of transition include a sense of well-being, mastery of the skills and behavior needed for success in the new environment, and well-being in the individual's personal relationships. Literature discussing outcomes of relocation is written with an almost exclusively pathogenic orientation. Relocation is viewed as something that can induce death and illness. This view is held regardless of the nature of the relocation.

Sense of Well-being

Lack of a sense of well-being, manifested by decreased life satisfaction, mood disturbance, morbidity or even mortality, has been associated with relocation among older adults. Perhaps the most disconcerting finding of some early studies was that relocation resulted in a increased mortality (Aldrich & Mendkoff, 1963; Bourestom & Tars, 1974; Pablo, 1977). However, mortality associated with relocation has been disputed (Borup, 1982; Borup & Gallego, 1981; Borup, Gallego, & Heffernan, 1979; Borup, Gallego, & Heffernan, 1980; Coffman, 1983; Grant, Skinkle, & Lipps, 1992; Markus, Blenkner, Bloom, & Downs, 1971; Ogren & Linn, 1971).

Mood disturbances such as depression (Anthony, Procter, Silverman, & Murphy, 1987; Johnson, 1992; Liebowitz, 1974), particularly in women (Dimond, McCance, & King, 1987), and increased aggression (Thomas et al., 1990) have been consistently identified as a result of relocation, and declines in life satisfaction (Pino, Rosica, & Carter, 1978; Wells & Macdonald, 1981) and mental functioning (Dube, 1982; Rajacich & Faux, 1988; Wells & Macdonald) have been found. However, improvements in emotional (Eckert & Haug, 1984) and physical health (Engle & Graney, 1993), and in physical function also have been documented (Harwood & Ebrahim, 1992; Pablo, 1977). Also, a primarily positive interpretation of the meaning of relocation has been identified (Johnson, 1996).

Morbidity associated with greater use of PRN medications and increased pain levels accompanied by declining ADL functioning (Eckert & Haug,1984; Ferraro, 1982; Gallagher & Walker, 1990) have been found following relocation. Additionally, self-rated health was found to be worse after relocation, particularly in female subjects (Dimond, McCance, & King, 1987). Similarly, earlier findings indicate a negative effect on health (Amenta, Weiner, & Amenta, 1984; Borup, Gallego, & Heffernan, 1980).

Mastery of New Behavior

There has been a lack of research investigating mastery of new behavior needed for successful adjustment to relocation, and what influences the perception of mastery. However, Ryff and Essex (1992) studied 120 older women who relocated to retirement communities or senior citizen apartment complexes. They found that environmental mastery was predicted by how positively or negatively subjects felt they compared with others in their situation. Environmental mastery also was predicted by lack of fit between the expectations and reality of the new environment.

Challenges of the new environment were identified by Johnson (1992), who found serendipitously that among older religious nuns who were relocated within their retirement home, learning to use new elevators, learning different routes to familiar places, and finding new locations of announcement boards were sources of stress. This was the case even though prerelocation preparation had been conducted. Study is needed to clarify the extent to which environmental mastery determines successful adjustment to relocation and how environmental mastery may best be facilitated among relocating older adults.

Well-being of Interpersonal Relationships: Social Support

Relocation has been found to influence social support negatively, that is, the number and extent of interpersonal relationships. This negative influence has subsequently been found to impede adjustment to relocation. For example, Tesch, Nehrke, and Whitbourne (1989) found that among 40 older veterans who relocated, peer friendships were disrupted as a result of the relocation. Their findings indicated that older men who had more active social relationships prior to relocation were more negatively affected by the disruption in networks following relocation than those who had minimal social networks previously.

Similarly, in a study of all women, Johnson (1992) found that social support was negatively influenced by relocation. The lack of research investigating the effects of relocation on social support may be especially problematic given that presence of social support has been found to enhance health and well-being. This area will be explored further in the discussion about interventions that nurses may undertake to facilitate relocation transition.

INTERVENTIONS TO PROMOTE HEALTHY RELOCATION TRANSITIONS

Researchers have found that when older adults actively participated in the relocation process (making the decision to move, deciding where they will move, planning, preparing, readying belongings, actually moving, and settling into the new environment), their adjustment was more positive than in those who had less participation. Nurses may play central roles in helping older adults participate in each component of the process, insofar as this is possible.

Helping Older Adults Participate in
Relocation Decision Making

The importance of choice, the desire to move, and control in deciding to move and where to move have been discussed in much of the relocation literature (Ferraro, 1981; Schulz & Brenner, 1977; Tesch et al., 1989). The concept of "home" has been found to mean, to older adults, a place where they can exercise some, if not absolute, control (Ruttman & Freedman, 1988). Unfortunately, studies show that older adults frequently are not able to control or are not afforded control or choice in relocation decisions (Johnson et al., 1994; Reinardy, 1992). Perceived choice has been found to be greater when there is a small difference in attractiveness of the options and when greater time is taken during option selection (Harvey & Johnston, 1973). Too often relocation of older adults may be precipitous caused by loss of a significant other, or failing health and lessening ability to perform ADLs. In this situation, preparation and fostering social support may play an even more important role in facilitating the adjustment to relocation. However, even in the event of precipitous relocation, older adults should be pivotal in making the decision to relocate and where to relocate, insofar as they want to participate and that it is possible.

In some early research, Smith and Brand (1975) studied 75 older adults, 40 of whom had relocated voluntarily to a nursing home and 35 of whom had been involuntarily transferred from other nursing homes. Subjects who had voluntarily relocated had better adjustments to life in the nursing home during the 3 months after moving. Relocation was negatively correlated with life satisfaction in those who had been involuntarily moved from other nursing homes.

Other researchers' work supports the importance of decisional control in relocation (Armer, 1996). For example, Reinardy (1992) found that those older adults who had made the decision to relocate (only 49% of the sample) felt more positively toward the move, and that this had a positive influence on health status and the ability to perform ADLs. Older adults with adult children were not any less likely to make the decision to move than those with no children.

Simply participating in the decision to move may not be enough to facilitate a positive adjustment. Ryff and Essex (1992) found that careful selection of the new home was central to adjustment. It was particularly important that discrepancies were minimal between what older adults expected of their new homes, and the reality of the new environment.

Nurses can assist older adults who are willing and able to make decisions about relocation to investigate various housing options and to collect information about them so as to make an informed choice about their new homes. Visiting the prospective homes is important to ascertain what type of resources, programs, and supports are available, what rules of conduct apply (in the case of structured facilities such as retirement facilities, senior apartments and nursing homes), and to meet other residents to find out how satisfied they are with their new home. Caregivers of older adults who are cognitively impaired or otherwise unable to make relocation decisions will need the same information.

Statewide organizations to which retirement, assisted living, and senior apartment facilities and nursing homes belong can provide information about resident satisfaction, turnover, and strengths and weaknesses of the facilities. These can be identified through Area Agencies on Aging and the American Association of Retired Persons (AARP). Additionally, the AARP and the U.S. Department of Health and Human Services have brochures and pamphlets available to assist nurses who are helping older adults and their caregivers in making relocation decisions. Table 3.1 shows a selection of these information sources. These materials may facilitate the older adult's decision-making process concerning relocation.

Helping Older Adults Prepare for Relocation

Whether or not older adults choose to or are able to make relocation decisions, there is agreement among research findings that preparation for relocation is important in facilitating adjustment. There may be overlap between decision making and preparation in that strictly speaking, the older adult will, by deciding to relocate, begin mentally preparing to relocate. Preparation can take many forms from making multiple visits to the new home, sampling the food, and reviewing menus (if food service is included), to meeting new neighbors before moving, clarifying what activities and services exist near or in the new location, and determining what personal possessions to move and liquidating the rest. Pino et al., (1978) studied 100 older adults who were relocated involuntarily. Four groups of participants were formed who were newly institutionalized: those who were prepared to move within the same institution, those who were not prepared, and finally those who did not move. Extent of participant preparation and involvement in decision making was considerable. Older adults in the prepared group selected their rooms and roommates. They participated

Table 3.1 Housing Resources Beneficial for Nurses and Older Adults

American Association of Retired Persons (AARP) Resources

"Facts About Older Women: Housing and Living Arrangements," a brochure providing statistics and information about housing costs.

"Housing Report," a periodic publication providing updates on housing issues, legislative initiatives, and the housing industry.

"Staying At Home: A Guide to Long-Term Care & Housing," a definitive source of information on evaluating housing options, also includes lists of additional resources.

"Understanding Senior Housing for the 1990's," a brochure providing findings of a recent study of 1,000 older adults regarding their housing preferences, concerns, and planning for their future housing.

These resources are available from AARP, Program Coordination and Development Department, 601 E Street, N.W., Washington, D.C. 20049.

Government Funded Publications

"Housing Highlights" is a series of factsheets on housing topics, including checklists to use in evaluating housing options, and additional resource information. Some of the more useful factsheets include "Assisted Living," "Government Assisted Housing," "Accessory Units," and "Shared Housing." These and other resources are available from the National Resource and Policy Center on Housing and Long-Term Care, USC Andrus Gerontology Center, 3715 McClintock Avenue, Los Angeles, CA 90089-0191.

---

in regular group activities in which they discussed their new facility and visited there before moving.

Prepared participants experienced fewer declines in ADLs and mental alertness than those who were unprepared. Participants who were institutionalized from community dwellings had greater decreases in life satisfaction, mental status, personality adjustment, and ability to perform activities of daily living than participants in any of the other groups.

Similar findings resulted from a study of 20 older adults who were relocated between institutions (Remer, 1986). Participants who were prepared showed less stress and greater life satisfaction following relocation than those who were not prepared. In a later work, Johnson and Hlava (1994) articulated preparatory interventions found beneficial in maintaining spirituality of older adults who relocated.

Liebowitz' (1974) participants experienced anxiety and depression when they were informed about impending relocation. The stress of the relocation may have been mediated by 1 week of preparation that included meetings to discuss the move, visits to the participants' new rooms, and one-to-one discussions with social workers. This preparation resulted in anxiety and depression levels returning to baseline 2 weeks after relocation.

Amenta, Weiner, and Amenta (1984) initiated a preparation program for participants moving from one nursing home to another in their study, which began with minimizing rumor by making the announcement of relocation in writing and during a resident's meeting 7 months prior to the actual move. They showed a film strip introducing the new facility and answered questions, and had staff members of the new facility visit the old facility to meet the residents. They also took the physically and mentally able older adults who were moving to visit the new facility on several occasions. Detailed profiles were developed on those who were moving (including physical, mental, and social status), and inventories were made of each resident's personal possessions. Three months prior to relocation, a designated staff member of the new facility met with each relocating resident to discuss their needs, desires, and concerns and to help them select possessions to bring to their new facility. Orientation booklets were distributed to relocating residents prior to their moving to provide them with information about their new facility. In addition, relocating residents were able to select their own roommates for the new facility.

Residents already living in the new facility were able to meet the new residents during their visits prior to moving. They also were given the option of moving within their facility and accepting new residents as roommates. Moving took place during a 2-week period. Once moved, the new residents had the option of participating in a wide array of activities and services. The study findings suggest that this type of preparation program was beneficial in improving the older adults' social activities, self-esteem, and personal care of themselves, areas that declined among those who did not relocate.

Participants in Walker and Gallagher's (1990) study were exposed to a similar program of preparation; however, the continuity of care was emphasized for older adults moving between extended care facilities. Another form of preparation, which Harwood and Ebrahim (1992) found to be beneficial was including older adults' family members in preparing for relocation by holding meetings to discuss the purpose and process of the relocation, by visiting new facilities, and by helping their older relative to pack and unpack belongings during the move. The staff of the nursing units also encouraged the older adults who were relocating to select color schemes, curtains, and furniture for their new nursing unit.

Related to this type of preparation is the necessity of sorting personal belongings, determining which ones will move to the new home, liquidating the rest, and packing. Loss of belongings has been found to be of concern to relocating older adults (Grant et al., 1992). Having continuity in assistance (one helper) with these tasks has been found to be beneficial during relocation (Johnson, 1992). Fewer helpers with packing may lessen the anxiety of being unable to find belongings when they are needed, being uncertain whether a particular item was liquidated or moved, and feeling overwhelmed with the prospect of unpacking in the new home. Nurses can help older adults identify their helpers for this challenging activity and encourage the helpers to remain committed to helping throughout the relocation process. Additionally, assisting the relocating older adult and the helpers to focus on what items can be taken to the new home rather than on what it is impossible to take may facilitate the relocation as a positive experience.

Thus the central components of preparation appear to be (1) giving information, (2) assessing the new environment, (3) having the option of exercising control in the process of relocation, (4) involving family members and friends insofar as this is possible and desired by the relocating older adult, and (5) visiting the new environment. Ryff and Essex (1992) also emphasized the importance of positive self-affirmations and self-assessments of the relocating older adult, which are facilitated by others positively affirming and assessing them. Nurses can help relocating older adults by reinforcing their accomplishments throughout the relocation process (such as gathering information about the new home, sorting and preparing personal belongings, planning how their belongings will be settled in the new home, meeting new neighbors), thereby promoting positive affirmations of older adults. This may facilitate a positive expectation of the new home and the older adults' belief that they can adjust and be happy in their new home. Thus one goal of preparation is minimizing discrepancies between relocating older adults' expectations of the new environment, their beliefs about their ability to thrive there, and the reality of the new environment.

While many of the components of this type of preparation best apply to relocation among older adults without cognitive impairment, involvement of family members and friends of confused older adults may be even more important. In parallel, where continuity of helpers is advisable among noncognitively impaired older adults, this may be especially important to minimize the stress of relocation among those who are cognitively impaired. Among these older adults, maintaining continuity of care as much as possible and ensuring that familiar objects and daily patterns are minimally disrupted or are readily restored to prerelocation patterns may be essential.

Bolstering the Well-Being of Interpersonal Relationships

A voluminous literature base discusses the benefits of interpersonal relationships in the form of social support of older adults in daily life, promoting health and well-being. Social interaction and support have been found to facilitate adjustment to relocation (Armer, 1996). Among rural older adults who relocated, availability of same-aged peers and support from family members were identified as instrumental in adjustment (Armer).

Similarly, Cohen, Teresi, and Holmes (1985) reported that the presence of social networks influenced the ability of older hotel residents to meet their physical, mental health, and physical self-maintenance needs. In this longitudinal research, social networks had both direct and buffering effects on the participants' ability to meet their needs. That is, the networks helped prepare the participants for stressful events and also helped them cope with the event while it was occurring and afterward. Structural characteristics of the networks (size, density, number of clusters, and configuration) were helpful predictors of ability to meet one's needs, especially among participants experiencing higher stress levels.

Previously, Wells and Macdonald (1981) found that the number and stability of close interpersonal relationships outside of the nursing home helped to minimize the negative effects of relocation between nursing homes. Other researchers have found extent and quality of social support networks to predict presence of depressive symptoms (Cutrona & Russell, 1987; Holahan & Holahan, 1987), and that the most prevalent means of coping was seeking social support in a group of older participants who had moved many times during previous years (Meeks, Carstensen, Tamsky, Wright, & Pellegrini, 1989).

Other research has demonstrated that social support helps older adults cope with life stressors, avoid illness, and live longer (Berkman, 1983; Blazer, 1982; Mor-Barak, Miller, & Syme, 1991). In fact, having at least one adult daughter or sibling has been found to reduce the risk of relocation to a nursing home (Freedman, 1996). Social support also has been found to influence the individual's self-perceptions, promoting well-being throughout the life course (Antonucci & Jackson, 1987; Kahn & Antonucci, 1980). These perceptions may then influence an individual's ability to respond to life stressors such as relocation. Social support also has been found to be an effective substitute for older adults' control over their environment in minimizing depression (Buschmann & Hollinger, 1994).

In contrast to research emphasizing the benefits of social support in adjustment to relocation, the findings of two studies do not concur. Tesch, Nehrke, and Whitbourne (1989) found that among older male veterans, presence of peer confidants was not associated with morale following relocation. The nature of the sample (all male veterans, without well-developed social support systems) may have contributed to this finding. Thomasma, Yeaworth, and McCabe (1990) found that older adults who were relocated to a more dependent-supportive environment had more anxiety following the move. Declining health and functional ability may have contributed to this finding. Although in these instances social support was not necessarily beneficial for older adults who relocated, the importance of assessing social support seems warranted to determine whether it is a usual coping mechanism in this population.

Social support networks of older adults may be dominated by their children and other family members (Shanas, 1979) or may consist of predominantly neighbors and friends. Each member may provide a different type of support ranging from instrumental assistance with daily living to emotional support. Some degree of reciprocity between the older adults and members of the support network is likely, although actions performed by one may not be similar to those performed by the other (Wellman & Hall, 1986). Social networks of women tend to be larger and more complex, including more family members but also including a diversity of individuals with whom relationships can differ vastly (Antonucci, 1990). Awareness of these patterns may guide nurses trying to help older adults adjust to relocation.

Activities in the new home that enable older adults to reciprocate with members of their social network may help to retain the integrity of the existing network. Nurses should advocate for social activities that are meaningful from the older adult's perspective and are amenable to including family and friends in order to help minimize the "out of sight, out of mind" phenomenon. This may be particularly important in congregate housing settings where it has been found that older adults report fewer positive group and family events than in nursing homes (Lawton, DeVoe, & Parmelee, 1996). In these settings, because older adults are typically more functionally independent, they may be less apt to receive needed visits, assistance, or encouragement than in nursing homes.

Additionally, insofar as retirement communities, senior citizen apartment facilities, and nursing homes integrate events of the larger community into their schedules of activities (such as piano recitals, craft shows, theater productions), there is greater likelihood that residents will have interaction with nonresidents. This integration also may promote participation of members of the residents' usual social networks, thereby increasing interaction.

Fostering introductions and ongoing interaction between newly relocated residents and their new neighbors through casual events such as ice cream socials, special dinners, picnics, or planned trips may help expand existing social networks to include new friends. Formal efforts such as neighborhood or facility newsletters, telephone trees to provide daily conversations, "buddy" welcoming programs, or health education classes that include sharing of ideas also may be helpful. Including members of the existing social network in these activities may provide a "bridge" for the newly relocated older adult who is not yet established in the new home neighborhood. Readily available social activities and opportunities have been found to impact positively the adjustment to relocation (Armer, 1996).

Other interventions such as cognitive group therapy and guided imagery have been found to be helpful in improving cognition of frail, institutionalized older adults (Abraham, Currie, & Neundorfer, 1992). In addition, pet ownership (particularly dog ownership) has been found to buffer the impact of stressful life events (i.e., relocation) (Siegel, 1990), and progressive relaxation has been found to positively influence self-esteem (Bensink, Godbey, Marshall, & Yarandi, 1993). Relocation is generally viewed as a potentially stressful life event that may influence the self-esteem of older adults.

Similarly, group reminiscence therapy has been found to have a significant positive influence on depression, particularly in the younger old (ages 65–74 years) (Arean et al., 1993; Youssef, 1990). Particularly effective themes (favorite holiday, first pet, and first job) for eliciting reminiscences among women have been articulated (Burnside, 1993). Interventions aimed at preventing or minimizing depression may be particularly salient because depression has been associated not only with relocation (as previously discussed), but also with environment. In particular, LaGory and Fitzpatrick (1992) found that older adults living in less "age dense or low accessibility neighborhoods" were more likely to have depressive symptoms (p. 459).

These interventions warrant testing with relocating older adults to identify their potential effects on other variables such as anxiety, life satisfaction, and adjustment following relocation. Additional work is needed in testing these and other interventions in order for nurses to most effectively help older adults adjust to relocation.

IMPLICATIONS

Practice

Whether relocation occurs as a developmental, situational, or health-related life transition, it is necessary that nurses recognize that it may result in considerable stress for older adults. With this recognition comes the responsibility to carefully assess older adults experiencing relocation and to intervene appropriately to minimize stress and facilitate adjustment to relocation.

Likewise, it is the role of the nurse to assist older adults (and their families) who are contemplating relocation by promoting participation of the older adult in decision making surrounding relocation insofar as this is desired and possible. As decisions are made, it is necessary for the nurse to help older adults and their family members acquire the information needed to select the best possible new home.

Helping to minimize discrepancies between the older adult's expectation and the reality of the new home may be an important facilitator of adjustment to relocation. Additionally, helping the older adult prepare for relocation, particularly with managing possessions, becoming acquainted with the new home, and promoting social support are also important interventions. Assistance with relocation transitions may be most effectively given when nurses are aware of the likelihood of appropriateness and success of interventions used.

Education

If nurses are to intervene effectively in facilitating older adults' adjustment to relocation, they must be made aware as students in basic and more advanced nursing education (particularly gerontic nursing education) of the potential for negative outcomes with relocation. Nursing home room transfers and relocation into different homes, retirement centers, senior citizen apartments, or nursing homes must not be viewed as inconsequential events for older adults. Careful assessment for relocation stress syndrome (RSS) is needed to guide nursing interventions. For example, according to NANDA (1996) selected defining characteristics for relocation stress syndrome include: change in environment location; anxiety; increased confusion; depression; loneliness; sleep disturbance; change in eating habits; dependency; increased verbalization of needs; and lack of trust. However, even in the absence of RSS, older adults may need assistance with decision making, preparation, and maximizing social support networks for relocation adjustment to occur. This content is a crucial component of nursing curricula.

Research

While the existing body of research is rich with explorations into the causes and effects of relocation for older adults, further empirical study is needed to test specific interventions aimed at smoothing relocation transitions and facilitating adjustment. For example, use of music, dance or art therapy, exercise, guided imagery, reminiscence, massage, cognitive therapy, structured information giving, and peer support need to be tested for their effectiveness. Nurses need to conduct this research, as it will further explicate their practice in the area of relocation of older adults.

Longitudinal studies are needed to identify the effects of relocation interventions over time. These are particularly needed because older adults tend to remain for relatively long periods of time between relocations. If they are slow in adjusting to their new homes, or if a particular relocation is viewed by them as unsuccessful, they may remain in need of nursing intervention. Thus nurses need to know the average length of adjustment time and effectiveness of interventions aimed at smoothing relocation transitions if older adults are to be assisted throughout the process of this potentially stressful experience.

REFERENCES

Abraham, I. L., Currie, L. J., Neese, J. B., Yi, E. S., & Thompson-Heisterman, A. A. (1994). Risk profiles for nursing home placement of rural elderly: A cluster analysis of psychogeriatric indicators. *Archives of Psychiatric Nursing, 8*(4), 262–271.

Abraham, I., Currie, L., & Neundorfer, M. (1992). Effects of cognitive group interventions on depression and cognition among elderly women in long-term care. *Journal of Women & Aging, 4*(1), 5–24.

Aldrich, C. K., & Mendkoff, E. (1963). Relocation of the aged and disabled: A mortality study. *Journal of the American Geriatrics Society, 11*(3), 185–194.

Amenta, M., Weiner, A., & Amenta, D. (1984). Successful relocation of elderly residents. *Geriatric Nursing, 5*(8), 356–360.

Anthony, K., Procter, A., Silverman, A., & Murphy, E. (1987). Mood and behavior problems following the relocation of elderly patients with mental illness. *Age and Ageing, 16*, 355–365.

Antonucci, T. (1990). Social supports and social relationships. In R. Binstock & L. George (Eds.), *Handbook of aging and the social sciences* (pp. 205–226). San Diego, CA: Academic Press.

Antonucci, T., & Jackson, J. (1987). Social support, interpersonal efficacy, and health. In L. Carstensen & B. Edelstein (Eds.), *Handbook of clinical gerontology* (pp. 291–311). New York: Pergamon.

Arean, P., Perri, M., Nezu, A., Schein, R., Christopher, F., & Joseph, T. (1993). Comparative effectiveness of social problem-solving therapy and reminiscence therapy as treatments for depression in older adults. *Journal of Consulting and Clinical Psychology, 61*(6), 1003–1010.

Armer, J. (1996). An exploration of factors influencing adjustment among relocating rural elders. *IMAGE: Journal of Nursing Scholarship, 28*(1), 35–40.

Barnhouse, A. H., Brugler, C. J., & Harkulich, J. T. (1992). Relocation stress syndrome. *Nursing Diagnosis, 3*(4), 166–167.

Bensink, G., Godbey, K., Marshall, M., & Yarandi, H. (1993). Institutionalized elderly relaxation, locus of control, self-esteem. *Journal of Gerontological Nursing, 18*(4), 30–36.

Berkman, L. (1983). The assessment of social networks and social support in the elderly. *Journal of the American Geriatrics Society, 31*, 743–749.

Blazer, D. (1982). Social support and mortality in an elderly community population. *American Journal of Epidemiology, 115*, 684–694.

Borup, J. (1982). The effects of varying degrees of interinstitutional environmental change on long-term care patients. *Gerontologist, 22*(4), 409–417.

Borup, J. H., & Gallego, D. T. (1981). Mortality as affected by interinstitutional relocation: Update and assessment. *The Gerontologist, 21*(1), 8–16.

Borup, J., Gallego, D., & Heffernan, P. (1979). Relocation and its effect on mortality. *The Gerontologist, 19*(2), 135–140.

Borup, J., Gallego, D., & Heffernan, P. (1980). Relocation: Its effect on health, functioning and mortality. *The Gerontologist, 20*(4), 468–479.

Bourestom, M., & Tars, S. (1974). Alterations in life patterns following nursing home relocation. *The Gerontologist, 14*, 506–510.

Burnside, I. (1993). Themes in reminiscence groups with older women. *International Journal of Aging and Human Development, 37*(3), 177–189.

Buschmann, M., & Hollinger, L. (1994). Influence of social support and control on depression in the elderly. *Clinical Gerontologist, 14*(4), 13–28.

Chick, N., & Meleis, A. I. (1986). Transitions: A nursing concern. In P. L. Chinn (Ed.), *Nursing research methodology: Issues and implementation* (pp. 237–257). Rockville, MD: Aspen.

Clifford, W. B., Heaton, T., & Fuguitt, G. V. (1982). Residential mobility and living arrangements among the elderly: Changing patterns in metropolitan and nonmetropolitan areas. *International Journal of Aging and Human Development, 14*(2), 139–156.

Coffman, T. (1983). Toward an understanding of geriatric relocation. *The Gerontologist, 23*(5), 453–459.

Cohen, C. A., Gold, D. P., Shulman, K. I., Wortley, J. T., McDonald, G., & Wargon, M. (1993). Factors determining the decision to institutionalize dementing individuals: A prospective study. *The Gerontologist, 33*(6), 714–720.

Cohen, C., Teresi, J., & Holmes, D. (1985). Social networks and adaptation. *The Gerontologist, 25*(3), 297–304.

Collins, C., King, S., & Kokinakis, C. (1994). Community service issues before nursing home placement of persons with dementia. *Western Journal of Nursing Research, 16*(1), 40–56.

Colsher, P. L., & Wallace R. B. (1990). Health and social antecedents of relocation in rural elderly persons. *Journal of Gerontology, 45*(1), S32–S38.

Cutrona, C, & Russell, D. (1987). *Social support and depressive symptoms among the elderly: A longitudinal causal modeling analysis.* Unpublished manuscript, University of Iowa, Iowa City, IA.

Dimond, M., McCance, K., & King, K. (1987). Forced residential relocation: Its impact on the well-being of older adults. *Western Journal of Nursing Research, 9*(4), 445–464.

Dube, A. (1982). The impact of moving a geriatric population: Mortality and emotional aspects. *Journal of Chronic Disease, 35*(1), 61–64.

Dunn, J. E., Furner, S. E., & Miles, T. P. (1993). Do falls predict institutionalization in older persons? *Journal of Aging and Health, 5*(2), 194–207.

Eckert, J., & Haug, M. (1984). The impact of forced residential relocation on the health of the elderly hotel dweller. *Journal of Gerontology, 39*(6), 753–755.

Engle, V., & Graney, M. (1993). Stability and improvement of health after nursing home admission. *Journal of Gerontology, 48*(1), S17–S23.

Ferraro, K. (1981). Relocation desires and outcomes among the elderly: A longitudinal analysis. *Research on Aging, 3*(2), 166–181.

Ferraro, K. (1982). The health consequences of relocation among the aged in the community. *Journal of Gerontology, 38*(1), 90–96.

Flynn, C. B., Longino, C. F., Wiseman, R. F., & Biggar, J. (1985). The redistribution of America's older population: Major national migration patterns for three census decades, 1960–1980. *The Gerontologist, 25*(3), 292–296.

Freedman, V. (1996). Family structure and the risk of nursing home admission. *Journal of Gerontology, 51B*(2), S61–S69.

Freedman, V. A., Berkman, L. F., Rapp, S. R., & Ostfeld, A. M. (1994). Family networks: Predictors of nursing home entry. *American Journal of Public Health, 84*(5), 843–845.

Gallagher, E. M., & Walker, G. (1990). Vulnerability of nursing home residents during relocations and renovations. *Journal of Aging Studies, 4*(1), 31–46.

Goetz, C. G., & Stebbins, G. T. (1994). Risk factors for nursing home placement in advanced Parkinson's disease. *Neurology, 43*, 2227–2229.

Grant, P., Skinkle, R., & Lipps, G. (1992). The impact of an interinstitutional relocation of nursing home residents requiring a high level of care. *The Gerontologist, 32*(6), 834–842.

Haas, W. H., & Serow, W. J. (1993). Amenity retirement migration process: A model and preliminary evidence. *The Gerontologist, 33*(2), 212–220.

Hallewell, C., Morris, J., & Jolley, D. (1994). The closure of residential homes: What happens to residents. *Age and Ageing, 23*, 158–161.

Harvey, J., & Johnston, S. (1973). Determinants of the perception of choice. *Journal of Experimental and Social Psychology, 9*, 164–179.

Harwood, R., & Ebrahim, S. (1992). Is relocation harmful to institutionalized elderly people? *Age and Ageing, 21*(1), 61–66.

Holahan, C. K., & Holahan, C J. (1987). Self–efficacy, social support and depression in aging: A longitudinal analysis. *Journal of Gerontology, 42*, 65–68.

Johnson, R. A. (1992). *Account-making and the meaning of translocation for elders.* Unpublished doctoral dissertation, University of Iowa, Iowa City.

Johnson, R. A. (1996). The meaning of relocation among elderly religious sisters. *Western Journal of Nursing, 18*(2), 172–185.

Johnson, R. A., & Hlava, C. (1994). Translocation of elders: Maintaining the spirit. *Geriatric Nursing, 15*(4), 209–212.

Johnson, R. A., Schwiebert, V. B., & Alvarado Rosenmann, P. (1994). Factors influencing nursing home placement decisions. *Clinical Nursing Research, 3*(3), 269–281.

Kahn, R., & Antonucci, T. (1980). Convoys over the life course: Attachment, roles, and social support. *Life-Span Development and Behavior, 3*, 253–286.

LaGory, M., & Fitzpatrick, K. (1992). The effects of environmental context on elderly depression. *Journal of Aging and Health, 4*(4), 459–479.

Lawton, M., DeVoe, R., & Parmelee, P. (1995). Relationship of events and affect in the daily life of an elderly population. *Psychology and Aging, 10*(3), 469–477.

Liebowitz, B. (1974). Impact of intra-institutional relocation. Special report from the Philadelphia Geriatric Center: Background and the planning process. *The Gerontologist, 14*(4), 293–295.

Litwak, E., & Longino, C. (1987). Migration patterns among the elderly: A developmental perspective. *The Gerontologist, 27*(3), 266–272.

Lord, S. R. (1994). Predictors of nursing home placement and mortality of residents in intermediate care. *Age and Ageing, 23* (6), 499–504.

Markus, E., Blenkner, M., Bloom, M., & Downs, T. (1971). The impact of relocation upon mortality rates of institutionalized aged persons. *Journal of Gerontology, 26*(4), 537–541.

Meeks, S., Carstensen, L., Tamsky, B., Wright, T., & Pellegrini, D. (1989). Age differences in coping: Does less mean worse? *International Journal of Aging and Human Development, 28*(2), 127–140.

Montgomery, R. J., & Kosloski, K. (1994). A longitudinal analysis of nursing home placement for dependent elders cared for by spouses vs. adult children. *Journal of Gerontology, 49*(2), S62–S74.

Mor-Barak, M., Miller, L., & Syme, L. (1991). Social networks, life events and health of the poor, frail elderly: A longitudinal study of the buffering versus the direct effect. *Family Community Health, 14*(2), 1–13.

Murtaugh, C. M., Kemper, P., & Spillman, B. C. (1990). The risk of nursing home use in later life. *Medical Care, 28*(10), 952–962.

Ogren, E., & Linn, M. (1971). Male nursing home patients: Relocation and mortality. *Journal of the American Geriatrics Society, 19*(3), 229–239.

Osterweil, D., Martin, M., & Syndulko, K. (1995). Predictors of skilled nursing placement in a multilevel long-term care facility. *Journal of the American Geriatrics Society, 43*(2), 108–112.

Pablo, R. Y. (1977). Intra-Institutional relocation: Its impact on long-term care patients. *The Gerontologist, 17*(5), 426–435.

Pino, C. J., Rosica, L. M., & Carter, T. J. (1978). The differential effects of relocation on nursing home patients. *The Gerontologist, 18*(2), 167–171.

Rajacich, D., & Faux, S. (1988). The relationship between relocation and alterations in mental status among elderly hospitalized patients. *Canadian Journal of Nursing Research, 20*(4), 31–42.

Reinardy, J. 1992). Decisional control in moving to a nursing home: Post admission adjustment and well-being. *The Gerontologist, 32*(1), 96–103.

Remer, D., & Buckwalter, K. (1990). Decreasing relocation stress for the elderly. *Continuing Care, 9*(9), 26–27, 42, 50.

Remer, D. (1986). *The effect of discharge preparation on the relocation of geripsychiatric patients.* Unpublished master's thesis, University of Iowa, Iowa City.

Ruttman, D., & Freedman, J. (1988). Anticipating relocation: Coping strategies and the meaning of home for older people. *Canadian Journal on Aging, 7*(1), 17–30.

Ryff, C. D., & Essex, M. J. (1992). The interpretation of life experience and well-being: The sample case of relocation. *Psychology and Aging, 7*(4), 507–517.

Schulz, R., & Brenner, G. (1977). Relocation of the aged: A review and theoretical analysis. *Journal of Gerontology, 32*(3), 323–333.

Schumacher, K. L., & Meleis, A. I. (1994). Transitions: A central concept in nursing. *IMAGE: Journal of Nursing Scholarship, 26*(2), 119–127.

Serow, W. (1987). Determinants of interstate migration: Differences between elderly and nonelderly movers. *Journal of Gerontology, 42*(1), 95–100.

Shanas, E. (1979). Social myth as hypothesis: The case of the family relations of old people. *The Gerontologist, 19*(1), 3–9.

Siegel, J. (1990). Stressful life events and use of physician services among the elderly: The moderating role of pet ownership. *Journal of Personality and Social Psychology, 58*(6), 1081–1086.

Smith, R., & Brand, F. (1975). Effects of enforced relocation on life adjustment in a nursing home. *International Journal of Aging and Human Development, 6*(3), 249–259.

Speare, A., & Meyer, J. (1988). Types of elderly residential mobility and their determinants. *Journal of Gerontology, 43*(3), S74–S81.

Speare, A., Avery, R., & Lawton, L. (1991). Disability, residential mobility, and changes in living arrangements. *Journal of Gerontology, 46*(3), S133–S142.

Tesch, S., Nehrke, M., & Whitbourne, S. (1989). Social relationships, psychosocial adaptation and intrainstitutional relocation of elderly men. *The Gerontologist, 29*(4), 517–523.

Thomas, M., Ekland, E., Griffin, M., Hagerott, R., Leichman, S., Murphy, H., & Osborne, O. (1990). Intrahospital relocation of psychiatric patients and effects on aggression. *Archives of Psychiatric Nursing, 4*(3), 154–160.

Thomasma, M., Yeaworth, R., & McCabe, B. (1990). Moving day: Relocation and anxiety in institutionalized elderly. *Journal of Gerontological Nursing, 16*(7), 18–24.

Uhlenberg, P. (1995). A note on viewing functional change in later life as migration. *The Gerontologist, 35*(4), 549–552.

Walker, S., & Gallagher, E. (1990). Environmental change and disruption in an extended care setting: Implications for the nursing role. *Perspectives, 14*(1), 6–12.

Wellman, B., & Hall, A. (1986). Social networks and social support: Implications for later life. In V. Marshall (Ed.), *Later life: The social psychology of aging* (pp. 191–231). Beverly Hills: Sage.

Wells, L., & Macdonald, G. (1981). Interpersonal networks and post-relocation adjustment of the institutionalized elderly. *The Gerontologist, 21*(2), 177–183.

Wolinsky, F. D., Callahan, C. M., Fitzgerald, J. F., & Johnson, R. J. (1993). Changes in functional status and the risks of subsequent nursing home placement and death. *Journal of Gerontology, 48*(3), S93–S101.

Yee, W., & Van Arsdol, M. (1977). Residential mobility, age, and the life cycle. *Journal of Gerontology, 32*(2), 211–221.

Young, J. E., Forbes, W. F., & Hirdes, J. P. (1994). The association of disability with long-term care institutionalization of the elderly. *Canadian Journal on Aging, 13*(1), 24–29.

Youssef, F. (1990). The impact of group reminiscence counseling on a depressed elderly population. *Nurse Practitioner, 15*(4), 32–37.

CHAPTER 4

Relocating Elderly Persons With Dementia: The Experience of Special Care Units

Janet P. Specht, Patricia T. Riley, Meridean L. Maas, David Reed, Lisa Skemp-Kelley, and Debra Schutte

Relocation of elderly persons with dementia is a fairly common event. This chapter focuses on the experience of nursing home Special Care Units (SCUs) for these individuals. Relocations, moves from one place of residence to another, occur when persons are first admitted to the SCU, when there is an acute health problem requiring hospitalization, when residents' conditions are no longer considered appropriate for the SCU, when needs can be better met on a different unit, or when finances are exhausted and the residents have to "go on" Title 19. Although there is substantial agreement that relocation has adverse effects on persons with dementia and their family caregivers, little research has been reported.

Issues addressed in this chapter include the effects of relocation on older persons, reasons for relocation, and the effects of relocation on SCU residents and their families. Possible strategies to promote healthy relocation of older persons and persons with dementia on SCUs are described. Finally, implications of relocation for clinicians, policy makers, nursing facilities, and research are discussed.

RELOCATION OF ELDERLY

Relocation has been shown to be potentially detrimental to both the physical and mental well-being of elderly persons, as described in the previous chapter. Yet change in physical environment is a common phenomenon for older persons as they make the transition from work to retirement, from marriage to widowhood, and from their family homes to living arrangements that are more manageable for their health and financial situations (Brand & Smith, 1974). Relocation is associated with chronic diseases, changes in functional abilities, cognitive impairment, falls, psychiatric illnesses, and changes in financial status (Engle, 1986). If older persons' health and functional abilities decline, they often face relocation to a hospital or nursing home (see Johnson, chap. 3 of this volume). These relocations can be temporary (when they are hospitalized) or permanent (when they move to sheltered housing or nursing homes). Thus relocations may be interinstitutional or intrainstitutional: interinstitutional relocations occur between settings, such as home to nursing home, while intrainstitutional relocations occur within settings, from one room to another or between units.

STRATEGIES TO MINIMIZE THE EFFECTS
OF RELOCATION ON ELDERLY PERSONS

Older persons perceive relocation as a stressful life event because of the changes in daily routines and social support that occur as a result of placement into their new locations (Johnson, chap 3; Stokes & Gordon, 1988).

Researchers have identified a number of effective modifiers in decreasing the detrimental effects of relocation. The degree of environmental change is one modifier of the response to relocation. Intrainstitutional or interinstitutional relocations are less disruptive than relocations from a home environment (Johnson, chap. 3; Mirotznik & Lombardi, 1995). Other modifiers of relocation include:

1. quality of the previous living environment;
2. resident's preparation for relocation;
3. whether the relocation was voluntary or involuntary;
4. age;

5. anticipated length of stay; and
6. number of relocations (Carp, 1967; Engle, 1985a, 1986; Lewis, Cretin, & Kane, 1985; Mirotznik & Ruskin, 1985; Reinardy, 1995).

An individual's older age and multiple transfers increase the negative consequences of relocation. When the relocation is to a better environment, or when the older person views the relocation as a short-term, rehabilitative move, there seem to be fewer adverse effects.

Duncan and Morgan (1994) focused on the effects of relocation on the families of older persons. Family members expressed concern about frequent relocation of their loved ones and its effect on relationships with staff. Family and staff relationships were perceived by families as vital to the care of residents. Relocation often necessitates establishment of new relationships with new staff caregivers after the move. However, little research is reported that has examined the effects of relocation on family members.

Armer (1993) identifies four research-based strategies for maximizing relocation adjustment. They are: (1) enhancement of perceived choice; (2) provision of opportunities for seeing the move as an option or a challenge rather than a threat; (3) increased predictability of the new environment; and (4) social support. Rajacich and Faux (1988) found that electively hospitalized elderly patients experienced less disorientation and confusion when they were part of the decision-making process. These elderly patients were admitted from noninstitutionalized settings for their surgeries and were given the opportunity to prepare for their admission. The preparation allowed the patients more time to orient themselves for the relocation. When people have more decisional control about relocation, they usually view the move more positively (Cox, 1996; Rajacich & Faux). Maintaining a positive outlook also is important in relocation. Focusing on the new location not as a place to die, but rather as an improvement over the old situation, may help residents adjust (Mirotznik & Ruskin, 1985).

Easing persons into a new situation and environment has better long-term outcomes than an unexpected change (Engel, 1985b). Methods for accomplishing this include (1) maintaining similar environments through placement of familiar furniture and personal belongings; (2) making several site visits prior to relocation; (3) ensuring resident's participation in packing and in choosing a roommate; (4) continuing personal routines (e.g., time of rising, bathing, manner of dress); and (5) providing information and facilitating maintenance of social support networks for residents and their families (Amenta, Weiner, & Amenta, 1984; Bellin, 1990;

Buschmann & Hollinger, 1994; Cohen, Teresi, & Holmes, 1985; Engle, 1985b; Johnson, chap 3; Mirotznik & Ruskin, 1985). Nurses are critical agents during the relocation and transition period and can facilitate the move by providing information as well as maintaining consistency for the family and new resident and being the familiar face for the resident during the transition. The more involved residents are with the relocation, the greater the likelihood of positive outcomes following the move.

RELOCATION OF OLDER PERSONS WITH DEMENTIA ON SCUS

SCUs for persons with dementia were developed in nursing homes in response to difficult care problems. Problems of ensuring safety on traditional, integrated units resulting from resident wandering, elopement, agitation, and altercations with other residents prompted the design of SCUs. SCUs were developed—many based on the Progressively Lowered Stress Threshold Model (Hall & Buckwalter, 1987)—to control environmental stimuli that were thought to often exceed the abilities of persons with dementia to process stimuli, thus resulting in increased stress and agitation. Although SCUs vary greatly, there is a consensus that five features are necessary:

1. admission of residents with dementia, most often Alzheimer's disease (AD);
2. specific staff qualifications and staff-resident ratios, selection, and training;
3. activity programming tailored for residents with dementia;
4. family programming and involvement in care; and
5. a segregated and modified physical and social environment (Maas, Swanson, Specht, & Buckwalter, 1994).

Admission and discharge policies are other common features of SCUs. These criteria are established in concert with the treatment goals, programming, and staffing plans of the SCUs. If the primary treatment goal of the unit is to provide a living area where ambulatory patients can safely wander, nonambulatory residents are not appropriate for the unit. Staffing ratios may be very different for persons who are ambulatory and require prompting and supervision compared to residents who require total assistance with daily care. Admission and discharge criteria are defined to ensure that SCUs provide the services for which they are established. However, these criteria also may result in the relocation of residents as their conditions change.

Little is reported about relocation of persons with dementia from SCUs, the effect of the relocation on their health and well-being, or the impact of relocation on their families. Since the ability to adapt to change involves an understanding of the situation, persons with dementia are particularly vulnerable to readjustment trauma following relocation (Damon, 1982). There is usually a 2-week adjustment period for newly relocated residents to become assimilated into SCU programming (Peppard, 1991). This adjustment period should be anticipated and planned for when relocating a person with dementia.

Maas and Swanson (1992) and Sloane and Matthew (1991) conducted research that examined relocation of residents to and from SCUs. The reasons for relocation that were documented in their studies included (1) inappropriate placement; (2) behavioral difficulties; (3) resident no longer benefits from special programming; (4) resident is no longer ambulatory; (5) resident no longer takes food orally; (6) a change in financial status; (7) acute illness; and (8) family request. Policies governing relocation of SCU residents often codify these reasons for discharge.

Sloane and Matthew (1991) studied 31 dementia units and 32 comparison units in five states. Half of the comparison units were in for-profit facilities and half of the units were in nonprofit facilities. Thirty-two of the nursing homes did not have an SCU. From retrospective chart reviews, the authors estimated one discharge per month for every 15–30 beds occupied by a resident with dementia. Sloane and Matthew explain that the constancy of residents on SCUs is related to the stability of their medical conditions. SCU residents were frequently discharged to family members or other nursing homes, whereas non-SCUs discharged acutely ill residents to the hospital.

Sloane and Matthew (1991) reported a high number of residents discharged from SCUs in the first 3 months after admission. They suggest that 10% of the residents were discharged from SCUs because of inappropriate placement, in contrast to only 1% of residents discharged from comparison units. Generally, inappropriate placement was related to the residents' level of functioning: either the residents were at too high a level of functioning or their behavioral difficulties were beyond the scope of the unit. Data from 171 residents in a "Family Involvement in Care" (FIC) study (Maas & Swanson, 1992) were examined for rates of relocation from SCUs. Data were collected between April 1994 and December 1996 from SCUs in 14 facilities in Iowa and Wisconsin; 2 of the homes were for profit, 10 were not-for-profit, and 2 were public operated. The size of the units ranged from 10 to 60 beds, with a median size of 16. All 14 SCUs in the FIC study are designed to serve residents in the middle stages of AD and include key features to promote safety, allow freedom while wandering or exploring the environment, enable management of behavioral problems, and promote maintenance of the residents' remaining functional abilities.

All of the facilities had at least one resident relocation during the 32 months of data collection. Twelve of the facilities had one or two residents relocated, while in two facilities, four residents relocated. The mean number of months between admission to the SCU and transfer was 26. Some of the reasons for transfer were: (1) the resident no longer benefited from SCU programming; (2) the resident was no longer ambulatory by means of walking or using a wheelchair (including a fractured hip or results from a stroke); (3) the resident was no longer private pay; (4) the family preferred the resident to be in a nursing facility closer to their home; and (5) the family wanted a less expensive nursing home.

While relocation has its noted effects on residents, disruptive behavior has become a significant reason for transfer. The FIC study found the most frequent reason to invoke the behavior policy was that residents were being aggressive toward other residents. When residents' behaviors were too disruptive, their transfers were most often made to acute psychiatric facilities or, in Iowa, to a state mental health institution. Advanced stages of dementia causing physical decline was another important reason for relocation from the SCUs. When persons were no longer ambulatory, they were transferred to other units in the facility that were designed to care for more functionally disabled residents. Eleven of the 14 FIC units required persons to be able to walk independently, or at least with a mechanical assistive device, to remain on the unit. None of the 14 units in the FIC study were prepared to care for persons when they were acutely ill; therefore, those elderly persons with dementia were transferred to acute facilities. One of the 14 facilities had a subacute unit, so SCU residents were transferred there for intravenous fluids and other subacute treatments. When they were stable, the residents were returned to the SCU.

Keyser-Jones, Wiener, and Barbaccia (1989) suggest several possible reasons for relocations from SCUs to acute facilities:

1. lack of required treatments such as intravenous therapy;
2. physician convenience;
3. extensive care requirements;

4. family request for dying resident;
5. pressure by the administration; and
6. poor communication among the involved parties.

Resident and family resources also may affect the ability to remain on an SCU. Homes that offer specialized care to a particular population often are viewed as having a commitment to quality care not ascribed to by those serving a general mixed population. This in turn may make the public more willing to pay a higher price for the care (Mor, Banaszak-Holl, & Zinn, 1995). Consequently, SCUs often accept only private pay residents. However, 12 of the FIC units did accept residents on Medicaid.

Frequently, when residents reach the end or terminal stage of dementia, they are transferred to traditional nursing home units. Thus if older patients with dementia do not wander, do not require the wandering safety feature of the unit, cannot participate in organized group activities, require extensive intervention for ADLs, or no longer present behavioral difficulties, they are transferred from the SCU.

EFFECTS OF RELOCATION ON PERSONS WITH DEMENTIA

No studies were found that measured the effects of relocating persons from SCUs. Further, very few studies reported the effects of relocation on persons with dementia from any setting. Documented effects of relocation on persons with dementia include increases in incontinence, mood swings, disruptive behaviors, persistent passive and withdrawal behaviors, depressive symptoms, disorientation that persists for months, and weight loss, resulting in a decrease in self-care ability (Anthony, Procter, Silverman, & Murphy, 1987; Bellin, 1990; Caine, Lyness, & King, 1993; Duncan & Morgan, 1994; Kim & Rovner, 1996; Lander, Brazill, & Ladrigan, 1997; Nirenberg, 1983).

Intrainstitutional relocation, however, appears to have less deleterious effects on persons with dementia than home-to-institution or interinstitutional transfers (Lander et al., 1997). No adverse effects of relocation were noted when the move was to a place where more appropriate care would be provided (Haddad, 1981). Further, cognitive status made no difference in 1 year postmortality rates in a comparison study of 207 relocated and 353 nonrelocated long-term care residents (Pruchno & Resch, 1988).

Relocation of persons with dementia often is unsettling for families and staff caregivers. Family members often do not want their relatives moved to an SCU if they have been on another unit at the nursing home for a substantial period of time. Likewise, the FIC study (Mass & Swanson, 1992) found families were upset when administrators recommended residents move out of the SCU. This finding is consistent with Duncan and Morgan (1994), who noted the distress of families because relocation meant starting new relationships with a different staff. Similarly, staff members experience increased stress when they must start again in forming new relationships with residents and families.

While relocation from SCUs is not a frequent event for most residents, a few residents experience multiple moves. Multiple relocations make adjustment very difficult for the resident and family. Two examples of difficulties associated with multiple moves are selected from the FIC study.

One son reluctantly admitted his mother to a nursing home from his home where he had been caring for her. She had dementia. He noted that the decision to place his mother in a nursing home was worse for him than going to serve in the Vietnam War. Six months after she was in the nursing home, personal financial resources ran out and she qualified for Medicaid. This particular SCU did not accept Medicaid payments, so she could no longer stay. The son took his mother home. Within 2 months he was unable to continue caring for her at home and transferred her to a facility 30 miles from where he lived. He was able to pay private pay rates for a few months but again ran out of funds, causing a transfer for his mother to another unit at the nursing home that accepted Medicaid payments. In less than 1 year this woman relocated five times.

In another case, a husband, cared for at home by his wife for 10 years since diagnosis, was admitted to an SCU because of his uncontrollable behavior. His behavior continued to be unmanageable in the nursing home, with periods of aggressiveness to other residents and staff. Because of this behavior, he was transferred to a state psychiatric facility two different times within a year. Consequently, he experienced five relocations in less than a year. Both the family and the resident suffered negative consequences from the multiple moves. With each move, the resident became less responsive and more dependent in ADLs. In interviews, the wife expressed more anxiety about her husband's deteriorating condition and his multiple relocations. When he was in the psychiatric facility, she saw him less often and received very little information about his condition. In this situation, it became difficult to sort out the negative effects of relocation from the deteriorating effects of the disease. The wife felt the moves had accelerated the deterioration of her husband's condition. This example also illustrates how relocation can exacerbate behavioral problems in persons with dementia.

One SCU in the FIC study relocated three residents to a skilled unit because of illness or immobilization. The skilled unit staff found these residents more difficult to manage after their relocation because of increased agitation and disruptive behaviors. More stimulation and the unfamiliar surroundings of the skilled unit may have resulted in the increased catastrophic behaviors of the newly relocated residents. Although it is unlikely that relocation was the sole cause of unmanageable behaviors, it was most likely an important contributing factor in the negative behavior.

STRATEGIES TO MINIMIZE RELOCATION EFFECTS ON PERSONS WITH DEMENTIA AND THEIR CAREGIVERS

One of the best ways to minimize the negative effects of relocation is through prevention. Some relocations can be prevented, but others to and from SCUs are necessary and desirable. Possible strategies to prevent negative effects of relocation include (1) minimizing the number of unnecessary relocations, (2) programming to prepare for known relocations, and (3) providing support services for those family and staff going through relocations. When residents with dementia were gradually oriented to their new location by emphasizing normal environmental cues, there was a decrease in disorientation, incontinence episodes, and mood swings (Bellin, 1990). Studies of older persons in non-SCU settings suggest that similarities in environments decrease the level of anxiety and disorientation residents experience after relocation (Bellin; Peppard, 1991). This research suggests that maintaining consistency of environments is an important factor in preventing negative effects of relocation upon older persons, especially those with dementia.

The Four Rs of Adjustment

Reisman (1987) identifies what he calls the four Rs of adjustment: reassurance, routes, routines, and relationships with persons from work. He believes these strategies helped his father, who was diagnosed with dementia, move into and successfully adjust to a nursing home. Reisman describes marked routes that helped his father find his way around in the new environment; routines that helped his father establish behaviors through repetition and reinforcement; and previous relationships that helped his father establish relationships with staff and other residents. These strategies are comparable to those identified by Armer (1993) to assist older persons with relocation. The last of the 4 Rs, the relationship's intervention, illustrates the importance of the involvement of family in the care of persons with dementia throughout institutionalization (Maas & Swanson, 1992).

The number of transfers between long-term care (LTC) facilities and acute care settings is an important consideration in minimizing relocation effects. A reduction in transfers also reduces the level of confusion and disorientation in persons with dementia (Keyser-Jones et al., 1989). Nurses need to understand the effects of these relocations and should intervene to prevent the transfers, if possible. A comprehensive relocation plan involving all staff, residents, and family, as well as postrelocation follow-up diminishes the stress of relocation (Brugler, Titus, & Nypaver, 1993; Hepburn, Petrie, Peterson, & Van Loy, 1995; Holzapfel, Schoch, Dodman, & Grant, 1992). Testing a relocation plan with a sample of residents with cognitive, mood, or psychotic disorders and partitioning the effects by diagnoses supported the advantage of relocation preparation (Lander et al., 1997). With intensive premove preparation and follow-up, there were significantly fewer negative effects of relocation. Lander et al. documented no weight loss, increase in disorientation, depression, anxiety, or irritable behaviors in cognitively impaired residents who perceived premove preparation.

Visiting the New Facility Before the Move

Easing persons into the new environment with visits to the location prior to the move is an important strategy to minimize relocation effects. Residents begin to identify areas of importance, such as the bathroom and dining areas, and recognize staff caregivers. Recognition of care providers may help residents be more comfortable in new surroundings. Relocation to a facility that has similar environmental cues has been found to reduce the number of incontinence episodes and decrease the catastrophic and inappropriate behaviors that surface as a reaction to the new environment (Bellin, 1990).

A new trend occurring in the delivery of health care is the development of subacute units (Parsons, 1996). Hospitals and LTC facilities have developed special units devoted to subacute patients. Providing subacute treatment in nursing homes prevents unnecessary transfers to a hospital. Residents with dementia and their families remain in closer proximity to familiar staff and return more quickly to their previous and familiar setting. Many residents are transferred to an acute setting because the LTC facility has inadequate facilities and professional providers are not available for certain treatments. Providing that care to residents within the LTC facility eliminates an unnecessary transfer to a hospital and decreases confusion for both residents and staff. The provision of in-house care thus may be more cost-effective for the residents and the facility and more advantageous for residents by eliminating some of the confusing transition process. Finally, providing these services also may foster better communication between the LTC staff and the physicians. Better monitoring of residents' conditions without the need for relocation outside the facility also results.

Another new trend in LTC facilities is the establishment of palliative care units for persons in terminal stages of dementia. These areas provide comfort and appropriate treatments and also maintain the resident's dignity until death (Kovach, Wilson, & Noonan, 1996). This unit prevents the unnecessary and upsetting practice of transferring residents to acute care just prior to death. Families are often upset with relocation of the resident from the SCU because they view the move as a sign of hopelessness and defeat (Hamidi, 1997). Palliative units address this concern by offering another form of specialized care, with the goal of providing comfort and maintaining dignity. Palliative care in LTC facilities assists in maintaining consistency in the environment as well as the crucial staff-family relationships that Duncan and Morgan (1994) identified.

Another strategy, used by one of the FIC sites, is the establishment of adjacent units, with programming for middle stage dementia on one unit and for late stage dementia on the other. This approach addresses the dilemma of providing specialized programming throughout a deteriorating course of illness and minimizes relocation effects (Mistretta & Kee, 1997).

Another example from the FIC study illustrates how staff on one skilled care unit worked to negate the effects of relocation on three residents. Following relocation from the SCU to a general nursing unit, three residents with acute illness had increased behavioral problems, especially at mealtimes. The nursing staff and social workers placed the three residents near each other during mealtimes to maintain some familiarity in their surroundings. The residents apparently recognized one another, their behaviors became more manageable, and their health stabilized enough for a successful return to the SCU. The decreased stimuli and familiarity of the SCU environment also may have positively affected the residents' uncontrollable behaviors. Thus, for this facility, moving the residents back to the SCU was successful. The skilled care unit staff in the facility continues to experiment with moving other residents back sooner following acute illness (e.g., fractures, pneumonia). They closely monitor the residents' return to the SCU and have noted a quicker recovery than when residents were maintained longer on the skilled nursing unit. This staff experimented with relocation to better manage residents with dementia and are continuing this practice with other SCU residents. For this facility, relocation of each resident is determined individually, and certain strategies are used to mitigate the relocation process. While this short-term relocation is not appropriate for all persons with dementia, in this situation it reduced the negative effects of relocation and was beneficial to the healing process.

DISCUSSION AND SUMMARY

There are a number of possible alternatives to decrease the negative effects of relocation on elderly persons with dementia. While persons with dementia are limited in decision-making capacities, providing alternatives during relocation gives an opportunity for decision making that may not be entirely lost. Providing a choice encourages residents to be part of the life-changing decisions. Encouraging them to help decide what clothes and personal items to bring to their new home also may foster a healthy relocation experience.

Some relocations are appropriate and necessary for the benefit of residents and families. Relocations from SCUs also are necessary to maintain the specialized SCU programming for target populations. However, it is important to minimize unnecessary relocations and plan ways to ameliorate the negative effects. Armer's (1993) principles provide guidance in this regard, but may require modification for persons with dementia. Other ways to reduce the number of relocations include

1. conducting preadmission screening for SCUs to help ensure persons are appropriately placed;
2. changing reimbursement policies to ensure that persons without private resources have access to care on SCUs;

3. providing selected treatments that have traditionally required hospitalization, such as intravenous therapy, either within the same facility or on the SCU;
4. ensuring continuity of care with familiar staff through consistent assignments and minimal turnover;
5. providing opportunities for families to become acquainted and establish relationships with new staff prior to intrainstitutional moves; and
6. providing specialized programming on adjacent units for varying stages of dementia.

There is a need for research to evaluate systematically the effectiveness of nursing interventions for minimizing negative relocation effects on persons with dementia and their families. Further, there is a need to evaluate the effectiveness of alternative models of care to minimize the number of relocations for persons with dementia. Clearly, one valuable approach would be to examine the role that family members can play in assisting residents in their transition within long-term care facilities. It is most significant to acknowledge that gerontological nurses have the opportunity to develop and test strategies to minimize the deleterious effects of relocation on persons with dementia in SCUs. These effects appear to have the potential to positively affect all those involved: staff, family members, and, most of all, the residents.

REFERENCES

Aldrich, C. K., & Mendkoff, E. (1963). Relocation of the aged and disabled: A mortality study. *Journal of the American Geriatrics Society, 11*(3), 185–194.

Amenta, M., Weiner, A., & Amenta, D. (1984). Successful relocation of elderly residents. *Geriatric Nursing, 5*(8), 356–360.

Anthony, K., Proctor, A. W., Silverman, A. M., & Murphy, E. (1987). Mood and behavior problems following the relocation of elderly patients with mental illness. *Age and Aging, 16*, 355–365.

Armer, J. M. (1993). Elderly relocation to a congregate setting: Factors influencing adjustment. *Issues in Mental Health Nursing, 14*, 157–172.

Bellin, C. (1990). Relocating adult day care: Its impact on persons with dementia. *Journal of Gerontological Nursing, 16*(3), 11–14.

Bourestom, N., & Tars, S. (1974). Alterations in life patterns following nursing home relocation. *The Gerontologist, 14*, 506–510.

Brand, F. N., & Smith, R. T. (1974). Life adjustment and relocation of the elderly. *Journal of Gerontology, 29*(3), 336–340.

Brody, E., Kleban, M., & Moss, M. (1974). Measuring the impact of change. *The Gerontologist, 14*, 299–305.

Brugler, C. J., Titus, M., & Nypaver, J. M. (1993). Relocation stress syndrome: A patient and staff approach. *Journal of Nursing Administration, 23*(1), 45–50.

Burnette, K. (1986). Relocation and the elderly: Changing perspectives. *Journal of Gerontological Nursing, 12*(10), 6–10.

Buschmann, M., & Hollinger, L. (1994). Influence of social support and control on depression in the elderly. *Clinical Gerontologist, 14*(4), 13–28.

Carp, F. M. (1967). The impact of environment on old people. *The Gerontologist, 7*, 106–108.

Caine, E. D., Lyness, J. M., & King, D. A. (1993). Reconsidering depression in the elderly. *American Journal of Geriatric Psychiatry, 1*, 4–20.

Coffman, T. L. (1983). Toward an understanding of geriatric relocation. *The Gerontologist, 23*(5), 453–459.

Cohen, C., Teresi, J., & Holmes, D. (1985). Social networks and adaptation. *The Gerontologist, 25*(3), 297–304.

Cox, C. (1996). Discharge planning for dementia patients: Factors influencing caregiver decisions and satisfaction. *Health and Social Work, 21*(2), 97–104.

Damon, L. E. (1982). Effects of relocation on the elderly. *American Family Physician, 26*(5), 144–148.

Duncan, M. T., & Morgan, L. L. (1994). Sharing the caring: Family caregivers' views of their relationships with nursing home staff. *The Gerontologist, 34*(2), 235–244.

Engle, V. (1985a). Mental status and functional health 4 days following relocation to a nursing home. *Research in Nursing & Health, 8*, 355–361.

Engle, V. (1985b). Temporary relocation: Is it stressful to your patients. *Journal of Gerontological Nursing, 11*(10), 28–31.

Engle, V. (1986). Bridging the research gap between acute and long-term care of older adults. *IMAGE: Journal of Nursing Scholarship, 18*(4), 148–150.

Haddad, L. B. (1981). Intra-institutional relocation: Measured impact on geriatric patients. *Journal of the American Geriatrics Society, 29*(2), 86–88.

Hall, G., & Buckwalter, K. (1987). Progressively Lowered Stress Threshold Model: A conceptual model for care of adults with Alzheimer's Disease. *Archives of Psychiatric Nursing, 1*, 309–406.

Hamidi, E. (1997). Your turn: How do you determine when a resident of a Special Care Unit for dementia should be discharged from that unit? *Journal of Gerontological Nursing, 23*(2), 47.

Harwood, R., & Ebrahim, S. (1992). Is relocation harmful to institutionalized elderly people? *Age and Ageing, 21*(1), 61–66.

Hepburn, K., Petrie, M., Peterson, C., & Van Loy, W. (1995). A moving experience:

Reconfiguring a special care unit for Alzheimer's patients. *The Gerontologist, 35*(6), 831–835.

Holzapfel, S. K., Schoch, C. P., Dodman, J. B., & Grant, M. M. (1992). Responses of nursing home residents to intrainstitutional relocation. *Geriatric Nursing, 13*(4), 192–195.

Horowitz, M. J., & Schulz, R. (1983). The relocation controversy: Criticism and commentary on five recent studies. *The Gerontologist, 23*, 229–234.

Johnson, R. A., & Halva, C. (1994). Translocation of elders: Maintaining the spirit. *Geriatric Nursing, 15*(4), 209–212.

Keyser-Jones, J. S., Wiener, C. L., & Barbaccia, J. C. (1989). Factors contributing to the hospitalization of nursing home residents. *The Gerontologist, 29*(4), 502–510.

Killian, E. C. (1970). Effect of geriatric transfers on mortality rates. *Social Work, 15*, 19–26.

Kim, E., & Rovner, B. (1996). The nursing home as a psychiatric hospital. In W. E. Reichman & P. R. Katz (Eds.), *Psychiatric care in the nursing home* (pp. 3–9). New York: Oxford University Press.

Kovach, C. R., Wilson, S. A., & Noonan, P. E. (1996). The effects of hospice interventions on behaviors, discomfort, and physical complications of end-stage dementia nursing home residents. *American Journal of Alzheimer's Disease, 11*(4), 7–15.

Lander, S. M., Brazill, A. L., & Ladrigan, P. M. (1997). Intrainstitutional relocation: Effects on residents' behavior and psychosocial functioning. *Journal of Gerontological Nursing, 23*(4), 35–41.

Lawton, M. P. (1980). *Environment and aging.* Monterey, CA: Wadsworth.

Lewis, M. A., Cretin, S., & Kane, R. L. (1985). The natural history of nursing home patients. *The Gerontologist, 25*(4), 382–388.

Lieberman, M. A. (1961). Relationship of mortality rates to entrance to a home for the aged. *Geriatrics, 16*, 515–519.

Maas, M., & Swanson, E. (1992). *Interventions for Alzheimer's: Family role trials.* Rockville, MD: National Institutes of Health.

Maas, M. L., Swanson, E. A., Specht, J. P., & Buckwalter, K. C. (1994). A nursing perspective on SCUs. *Alzheimer Disease and Associated Disorders, 8*(Suppl. 1), S417–S424.

Mirotznik, J., & Lombardi, T. (1995). The impact of intrainstitutional relocation on morbidity in an acute care setting. *The Gerontologist, 35*(2), 217–224.

Mirotznik, J., & Ruskin, A. P. (1985, Winter). Interinstitutional relocation and the elderly. *Journal of Long-term Care Administration*, 127–131.

Mistretta, E. F., & Kee, C. C. (1997). Caring for Alzheimer's residents in dedicated units. *Journal of Gerontological Nursing, 23*(2), 41–49.

Moos, R. H., David, T. G., Lemke, S., & Postle, E. (1984). Coping with an intrainstitutional relocation: Changes in resident and staff behavior patterns. *The Gerontologist, 24*(5), 495–502.

Mor, V., Banaszak-Holl, J., & Zinn, J. (1995). The trend toward specialization in nursing care facilities. *Generations, 19*(4), 24–29.

Nirenberg, T. (1983). Relocation of institutionalized elderly. *Journal of Consulting and Clinical Psychology, 51*(5), 693–701.

North American Nursing Diagnosis Association [NANDA]. (1997). *NANDA Nursing Diagnoses: Definitions and Classification 1997–1998.* Philadelphia: North American Nursing Diagnosis Association.

Parsons, Y. (1996). Get with the subacute program. *Contemporary Long-Term Care, 19*(7), 64–67.

Peppard, N. (1991). *Special needs dementia units: Design, development and operations.* New York: Springer.

Pruchno, R. A., & Resch, N. L. (1988). Intrainstitutional relocation: Mortality effects. *The Gerontologist, 28*(3), 311–317.

Rajacich, D. L., & Faux, S. (1988). The relationship between relocation and alterations in mental status among elderly hospitalized patients. *Canadian Journal of Nursing Research, 20*(4), 31–42.

Reinardy, J. (1995). Relocation to a new environment: Decisional control and the move to a nursing home. *Health & Social Work, 20*(1), 31–37.

Reisman, B. (1987, March/April). Adjusting to a residential facility for older persons: A child's perspective. *American Journal of Alzheimer's Care and Research,* 37–42.

Sloane, P., & Matthew, L. (1991). *Dementia units in long-term care.* Baltimore: Johns Hopkins University Press.

Stokes, S. A., & Gordon, S. E. (1988). Development of an instrument to measure stress in the older adult. *Nursing Research, 37,* 16–19.

CHAPTER 5

Coping With Death: Grief and Bereavement in Elderly Persons

Richard H. Steeves and David L. Kahn

L oss is an inevitable part of aging. Much has been written about how elderly people respond to and recover from the losses associated with aging. The loss associated with the death of significant others is a major one and thus attracted the attention of many researchers. However, there is still not a mature body of research in this area. That is, no clear agreement exists regarding how to intervene to help people in their grief. In fact, writers in the area do not even agree that interventions are needed or helpful. This chapter focuses on the issue of grief and bereavement in elderly persons and the possibility of interventions to ameliorate the effects of such losses. The following discussion is divided into four sections. The first section presents what is known about bereavement and its effects on elderly persons. The second identifies the variables that affect the course of bereavement. The third is a review of the interventions that have been tested with bereaved elderly persons, and the final section is a recommendation including a new intervention to be tested.

BACKGROUND

Since the early studies by Parkes (1964a, 1964b, 1965, 1971) and Lindemann (1944), researchers have documented the effects of loss and grief on people, including older adults. These effects include both changes in morbidity and mortality. As might be expected, most of this research has focused on bereavement related to the death of a spouse. For example, Rogers (1995) found that marriage has a protective effect on people and widowed people were more likely to die at a younger age than their matched counterparts. Similar findings regarding mortality were described by Bowling (1988/1989).

Some researchers have concentrated on the physiological effects of bereavement. Jacobs (1987), for instance, studied changes in the endocrine system, including prolactin, growth hormone, cortisol, and epinephrine. He found changes in the level of all these substances in the early weeks of bereavement. While he could not discriminate between bereavement and other kinds of loss, Jacobs was able to establish the extent of the bodily response to grief. Irwin and Pike (1993) reviewed studies of immune function in bereavement. Taking depression as the mediator between immune indicators and bereavement, they presented evidence of "a reduction of in vitro correlates of cellular immunity" (p. 171). Reynolds et al. (1993) studied the sleep patterns of a sample of bereaved elderly people. Using multiple measures of sleep patterns, they discovered that the amount of time spent in REM sleep was increased during the first months of bereavement. Deep restful sleep was not as frequent, and dreaming was increased.

The majority of the research on bereavement in older adults has concentrated on psychosocial effects. Lund, Caserta, and Dimond (1993) provided a comprehensive list of the psychosocial effects of loss in their review of the research literature on bereavement in older adults. They noted that studies had documented problems with family relationships and friendships, confused personal identity, low self-esteem, anger, guilt, and depression as typical sequelae of loss.

Approaching the area of loss from different perspectives, a number of researchers have used multiple measures of general function and well-being to investigate the untoward effects of bereavement on older people. For example, Bennett (1996), noting that 65% of women above 74 years old are widowed, measured the mental and physical health of three samples of elderly women: never married, currently married, and widowed. Not surprisingly, she found age-related declines in physical health, morale, and social engagement, and a rise in personal disturbances across all three groups. However, over and above these changes, the widows did less well than the other groups in terms of personal disturbances and morale. Even though these indicators declined after the death and rose again in subsequent months in this 8-year study, for several years after the death of their husbands, the widows remained significantly different from the other elderly women on these measures.

Similarly, Byrne and Raphael (1997) found that widowers do not fare well after bereavement either. These researchers identified a group of men who had recently lost a spouse by using official death notices. The men were interviewed 6 weeks, 6 months, and 13 months postbereavement using a 22-item self-report instrument. A matched group of men who were still married were interviewed at similar intervals. Although no differences were noted in loneliness and depression, the widowers suffered from more state anxiety and general psychological distress than did the married men. The widowers also reported more sleep disturbances and more thoughts of death and suicide.

One major source of concern for researchers has been depression in the bereaved elderly. Pasternak et al. (1994) identified a group of elderly bereaved people who suffered from what they termed "subsyndromal depression." They followed 20 bereaved persons with depressive symptoms over a 2-year period and compared them to a nondepressed group of bereaved older adults and a group that was neither bereaved nor depressed. The group with subsyndromal depression had greater impairment of work and pleasure and more anxiety. Up to 2 years later, this group suffered from self-reported sleep disturbances and were rated lower in the amount of social support they received and in measures of general functioning than either of the other two groups.

In a 25-month study of bereaved widows and widowers, Zisook and Shuchter (1993) assessed rates of depressive symptoms and syndromes and morbidity associated with depression of widowhood. After determining the risk factors for major depression, they discovered that the single best predictor of major depression at 25 months was the presence of a depressive syndrome at 7 months. These researchers argue that although depressive episodes are not uncommon in spousal bereavement and are considered part of uncomplicated bereavement, these episodes are not benign and can lead to major depression later.

Another area of scientific interest and concern has been the social isolation of bereaved elderly people. In a review of her own work and the work of others in the field, Lopata (1993) concluded that older widows in urban America face numerous problems and have a high risk of becoming socially isolated. Lopata notes that in many of the studies she reviewed, urban widows were socialized in either ethnic communities in the United States or in village life in other countries. Because of the prevailing culture in America, according to Lopata's hypothesis, these women depended for support on primary relationships such as a husband, sisters and brothers, and eventually their children. Their husbands on the other hand were more engaged in public life and developed friendships and relationships outside the family. When the husband died, according to Lopata, the widow's life became disorganized and her major sources of support disappeared. She had a significant possibility of eventually living with a family member such as a married daughter and becoming socially isolated.

Using qualitative methods to study widowhood in a retirement community in Florida, van den Hoonaard (1994) questioned the assumption that retirement communities would be good places for widows to find the social support they need because of the homogeneity of age. Van den Hoonaard discovered that widows were second-class citizens in the community. Because they did not have husbands, they were not treated as equals by the married retired women in the community. The married retirees associated with other married couples and were not available for friendships with the widows. Status as a bereaved person was detrimental to the welfare of these widows who found themselves in limited circumstances with reduced social status.

THE LACK OF EFFECT OF BEREAVEMENT

Despite a growing body of literature like the previous example, the assertion that bereavement has serious and long-lasting deleterious effects remains controversial. Even the physiological researchers who have documented changes in the endocrine and immune systems in the first few weeks of bereavement have not established that these changes have long-lasting effects. In fact, the sleep researchers (Reynolds et al., 1993) demonstrated that normal sleep patterns returned for their bereaved subjects in 2 years.

Looking for the predicted decline in social integration in widows, Pellman (1992) interviewed 160 women 60 years old and older in the Kansas City area. Eighty of the women were widows and 80 were not. In addition to integration into the community, Pellman also was interested in stress, daily hassles, social networks, and support-seeking behavior. She discovered that age and education were better predictors of the variables than was widowhood. Daily hassles did not correlate with stress, and those elderly people who sought support were not the ones who needed it the most. She concluded that the effects of bereavement on older adults may not be as detrimental as believed and that demographic variables and aging have more effect.

In this same vein, Murrell, Himmelfarb, and Phifer (1995) studied the effects of the loss of a close significant other such as a spouse, the effects of the loss of a less significant other, and the effects of the loss of something like a house or business or pet on the health and general function of 50 elderly people. The researchers interviewed the participants at 6-month intervals for up to 2 and a half years. They reported that health actually improved after bereavement and the loss of a business, house, or pet had a more negative effect on health than did bereavement.

Similarly, Costa, Zonderman, and McCrae (1991) argued that although bereavement in older adulthood is painful and widowers and widows never forget their dead spouses, they do learn to accept the loss, and bereavement eventually has little effect on daily mood and functioning. Using a national probability sample in a 10-year study, these researchers measured self-rated health, ADLs, size of social networks, extroversion, openness to experience, psychological well-being, and depression. Surviving spouses showed little or no difference on these measures from men and women in intact families.

In another example, Matthews (1991) examined the experience of widowhood in later life for Canadians. She noted that the death of a spouse is still the most typical way for married life to end, but that in most research widowhood has been treated as a stressful and traumatic life event. Her research, however, demonstrated that widows generally adapted very well over time and widowed people generally had more functional supporters in their social networks than did divorced people.

It has been assumed that the death of a spouse starts widows and widowers on a general decline in their economic well-being. Zick and Smith (1991) investigated this assumption as an empirical question. Using data from an 11-year period, these researchers compared middle-aged and elderly widows and widowers to men and women in the same age groups living in intact families. Contrary to the standard hypotheses, the elderly widows and widowers began their economic decline 5 years prior to the death of their spouse. The sample of bereaved older adults in this study were different initially from the older adults in intact families. These findings suggested that those people who were widowed may have made different economic choices over their lifetimes than their counterparts who were in intact families. In Zick and Smith's study, economic status seems to have been a function of some other cause and not bereavement.

Given literature such as that presented in this section, it is not clear whether bereavement has serious long-term consequences or not. The most probable hypothesis is that bereavement is deleterious for some older adults, while others, still hurt by their loss, survive intact. If this is the case, then the problem becomes one of determining which bereaved persons are most at risk for lasting effects.

VARIABLES AFFECTING RESPONSE TO BEREAVEMENT

Much effort has been spent recently to identify and determine which variables increase the risk of harmful and lasting effects of bereavement in elderly persons. In an extensive review of the state of knowledge about bereavement and mental health in elderly persons, Parkes (1992) noted the importance of identifying high-risk bereaved people and identified a number of risk factors that contribute to poor outcomes: (a) the type of death—sudden loss was more difficult than death after a long illness, (b) poor health status, (c) a large number of previous losses, (d) having a close relationship with the deceased, and (e) lack of access to social support.

Other researchers also have compiled extensive lists of what they believed were important variables. For instance, Lund et al. (1993), using the data from two longitudinal studies, investigated the course of spousal bereavement in later life. They used a standardized measure of life satisfaction, two depression scales, and the Revised Texas Inventory of Grief, an often used tool in bereavement studies. Their findings indicated that bereaved spouses were diverse and the course of bereavement was not one of stages but rather "like a roller coaster ride of many ups and downs" (p. 247). Loneliness was the most often reported problem, and managing daily living skills was a chief difficulty especially for widowers. Eighty percent of the bereaved were managing satisfactorily after 2 years. According to Lund et al., the best predictors of good outcomes were (a) amount of time since the death (the passage of time makes life easier); (b) initial or early bereavement adjustments (doing badly at first was a good predictor of eventual management problems); (c) being able to communicate with others about thoughts and feelings; (d) positive self-esteem; and (e) personal competencies, that is, the ability to muster resources and adapt to new environments. Lund et al. were surprised to find that social support was not on this list of predictor variables.

Social Support

However, social support, as a variable that improves bereavement outcomes, has been verified in other studies. For example, taking depression as a preventable outcome of bereavement in elderly people, Prigerson (1993) studied a sample of 79 recently widowed older adults for approximately 1 year. His hypothesis was that three classes of psychosocial factors affect depressive symptoms: (a) social supports; (b) mastery events (i.e., events that promoted self-sufficiency and confidence); and (c) social rhythms (i.e., maintaining regularity and stability in one's social activities). Social support, more than the other variables, reduced the likelihood of being or becoming depressed after spousal loss. Mastery events were correlated with depression but did not seem to be effective in reducing the likelihood of dysthymia. Maintaining social rhythms did not have a significant effect on depression during the 1st year of bereavement.

A study by Willert, Beckwith, Holm, and Beckwith (1995) offered more arguments for the importance of social support. Forty-four, primarily elderly spouses of patients were assessed within 2 weeks after being admitted to a hospice. Several different types of social support and specific coping strategies were regressed on measures of depression, anxiety, anger, and physical symptoms. Findings indicated that specific types of social support, socialization, guidance, and cognitive information as well as the self-report of the coping strategy of wishful thinking were associated with anxiety. Also, cognitive information coupled with coping strategies of wishful thinking and expressed emotions were associated with anger. Interestingly, the authors do not report any effect of social support or coping strategies on depression or physical symptoms.

Social support appears to have an effect on mortality after bereavement in older adults. Bowling (1988/1989) wanted to know if there were variables that could be used to predict which of the bereaved were in the most danger of dying. Using population census data to recruit a sample of 503 elderly bereaved people in England whom he followed over time, Bowling identified five risk factors: male, 75 years old or older, depression or low happiness levels, high social class, and lack of social support. Bowling also concluded that having a close personal relationship is critical for psychological well-being in the bereaved elderly.

A number of researchers have looked not just at social support but at specific aspects of social interactions and how particular attitudes play into social support during bereavement. Ulmer, Range and Smith (1991) found that a sense of purpose in life, probably interacting with social support, made bereavement less difficult in their sample of 122 newly bereaved people (not all of whom were old). Aber (1992) also found that social support was significantly related to coping with bereavement, interacting with a longer work history and positive attitudes to work. Herth (1990) reported that social support, operationalized as the frequency of visits by family members, was significantly related to higher levels of grief resolution and hope, while a negative relationship was found between the level of grief resolution and the use of evasive, fatalistic. and emotive coping styles.

Prior Relationship

The relationship between the bereaved person and the one who has died has been the subject of much conjecture and some research. The widely held belief is that the closer the emotional tie to the loved one, the more difficult the period of bereavement (Leahy, 1992/1993; Sanders, 1979/1980). Chenell and Murphy (1992) demonstrated that if a relationship was more central or close, the level of symptoms during bereavement would be higher.

Anticipatory Grieving

Brouke (1984) reviewed the literature on the relationship between pre- and postbereavement grieving by exploring the assumption that anticipatory grief could act as a buffer to grief after the death. Many of the studies reviewed were conducted with older adults. Brouke found that the study results were mixed. Some showed that anticipatory grief increased the postdeath grief and other studies showed the opposite. His reasonable conclusion was that bereavement should be viewed as an ongoing experience. That is, predeath experiences should not be seen as variables affecting postdeath experiences, rather pre- and postdeath grief should be seen as different stages in the same process.

Another interesting study in this area is one by Kramer (1997). Although this was not specifically a study of elderly persons, the mean age of the widows in this study was close to 60 years old. Kramer cited the work of previous researchers, such as Lindemann (1944), who have argued that separation from a dying loved one before the death is not a positive step, and Glaser and Strauss (1965), who stated that it was vital that husbands and wives talk about the upcoming death openly. Kramer then showed, using the data from her own study, that the women who were realistic about the upcoming death of their husbands and began to separate mentally from them adjusted better to bereavement. In a separate finding, her data showed that the women who did not feel the need to discuss the upcoming death with their husbands also did better during the period of adjustment.

Circumstances of Death

Starting with early work by Parkes (1975/1976), some attention has been paid to the effect of the circumstances of death on the subsequent bereavement course. However, none of the research has been directed at an aged population specifically. In addition, many of the studies dealt with only short-term effects (Lehman, Ellard, & Myrick, 1986; Parkes & Weiss, 1983; Range & Thompson, 1987). Lehmand, Wortman, and Williams (1987) looked at long-term effects but only in the narrow case of death in automobile accidents. Range and Niss (1990) looked at a variety of circumstances of death over a long-term period but used only college students for subjects. Contrary to the other studies, Range and Niss found no relationship between bereavement outcomes and the circumstances of death. Clearly, it is too early to say anything conclusive about the circumstances of death and the subsequent course of bereavement in elderly people.

Mood

The research on mood as a predictor variable in relation to bereavement is not clear either. Hays, Kasl, and Jacobs (1994), in a prospective study of elderly persons who might become widowed, studied the effect of a previous history of dysphoria on aspects of bereavement. Spouses of patients undergoing elective surgery or hospitalized for serious illness were recruited, and over a 25-month period, during which a number of the subjects became widows, researchers used standardized instruments to measure depression, anxiety, hopelessness/helplessness, past history of dysphoric mood, and methods of coping. These researchers discovered that the bereaved with a history of previous dysphoria categorized their social networks as nonsupportive. However, compared to the subjects without a history of dysphoria, these subjects spent a similar amount of time in social interactions and in seeking support. Also, subjects with a history of dysphoria prior to the bereavement had higher rates of depressive symptoms, general anxiety, and helplessness/hopelessness. Yet, over the course of the study, the subjects with the history of dysphoria had similar recovery trajectories to those without a history.

Zisook and Shuchter (1993) also reported somewhat contradictory findings. These researchers attempted to enumerate the predictors of major depression during bereavement. They found that the best predictor of depression at 25 months after the loss of a spouse (the length of the study) was depressive symptoms at 7 months after the loss. In other words, an early response to the loss seemed to affect later recovery. Other significant variables also were identified: a family history of major depression was associated with postwidowhood depression, as were postbereavement alcohol consumption, prebereavement medical visits, and an unanticipated or sudden death of the spouse.

BEREAVEMENT INTERVENTIONS

There is a paucity of reports regarding designing and testing interventions for bereavement, as might be expected given the extant knowledge of effects and precise variables that might affect the course of bereavement for older adults. The interventions that have been and are being used generally fall into two categories: individual or group psychotherapy, and the provision of social support.

Psychotherapy for bereavement has been going on for some time, and it has taken all the forms that psychotherapy for other putative psychological problems has: Freudian, Jungian, existential, group and one-to-one. The methodological problems with evaluating the effectiveness of these different interventions are the same as with evaluation of psychotherapy in general. It is very difficult or unethical to randomize; and it is problematic to match in different groups because of the difficulty in identifying the variables that affect the outcomes of both bereavement and psychotherapy. Because the establishment and importance of the therapeutic relationship depends to some degree on the personalities of the therapist and the client, it is difficult to establish a standard delivery of the intervention.

Stern (1990), in a monograph considering psychotherapy and widowhood, informally surveyed approximately 200 practicing psychotherapists and discovered very few of them had widowed patients that had come to them specifically because their spouses had died. While most agreed that dependency issues had an effect on how well widows were able to develop emotionally, they also agreed that the negative effects of widowhood did not necessarily disappear with time.

Stroebe, Stroebe, and Hansson (1993) have edited the most complete resource on the treatment of bereavement to date. In that volume, Raphael, Middleton, Martinek, and Misso (1993) considered the intervention of counseling and therapy of the bereaved. These authors reviewed the research on grief therapy as a preventive intervention for the psychological and physical effects of bereavement and as a palliation for the pain of grief. After pointing out the problems with multiple definitions of grief, the lack of a clear description of interventions in many cases, and the variability in the outcomes measured, the authors, nevertheless, conclude that "there is much supportive evidence indicating that bereavement counseling is effective, both as a preventive measure for bereaved people who are at high risk and as a therapeutic intervention" (p. 452).

In the same volume, Lieberman (1993) reviewed the literature on self-help groups for the bereaved. Although he did not confine his review to studies of older adults, the means and medians he reported for the age of the subjects in the studies reviewed are at least in the mid-50s. Lieberman reiterated similar methodological problems to those with intervention studies previously discussed under the consideration of psychotherapy. He also noted the problem of the wide variety of views regarding the nature of bereavement and the "problem" that brought bereaved persons to self-help groups held by individual members of the self-help groups.

The studies reviewed by Lieberman used self-help groups that varied widely in settings and conditions, outcome measures, outcome measurement points, and criteria for subject inclusion. Lieberman identified three kinds of self-help groups in the studies:

1. existing groups of extended longevity that were established and controlled by the lay members;
2. short-term groups that were run by mental health professionals; and
3. groups established by the researchers for the study.

The outcome measures ranged from clinician ratings, to established questionnaires about symptoms, to written self-reports about roles and grief intensity. Lieberman reported that some of the studies were well done and others had serious sampling or measurement problems. He concluded that while there was some evidence that self-help groups could be helpful, the lack of consistency and variability among studies about conditions or settings and about the definition of self-help made it impossible to develop precise statements about the efficacy of self-help groups.

McKibbin (1997), dealing with a small sample in a pilot study and using a waiting list as a control group, demonstrated that self-help groups meeting for six sessions over a 3-week period could reduce psychological stress. McKibbin, who was most interested in locus of control, found that participation in a self-help group increased the desire for locus of control.

Caserta and Lund (1993) looked specifically at older adults who had been widowed and the effect of self-help groups. They looked at the duration of the self-help group and the three interpersonal resources of self-esteem, competencies, and life satisfaction. The outcome measures were depression and grief. Those older adults with low competencies did better (as defined by lower ratings of depression and grief) the more they attended the self-help groups. However, in the short term, older adults with high competencies reported a higher level of grief and depression after attending the self-help group sessions. These high readings seemed to resolve with long-term monthly attendance. Thus it seems that self-help groups are useful for people with certain characteristics, and, more importantly self-help groups may actually have negative consequences for some people. Obviously, this issue, particularly because of the latter possibility, needs more empirical investigation.

A THEORETICAL FRAMEWORK AND PROPOSAL

The theoretical work in the area of bereavement among elderly persons and in general is no more clear than is the empirical work. The earliest theoretical work emerged from the psychoanalytic traditions (Bowlby, 1980; Freud, 1917; Lindemann, 1944). The part of the psychoanalytic tradition that remains, for the most part, in current theory about bereavement is the idea of grief work (Raphael & Nunn, 1988; Rosenblatt, 1993). Grief work is the notion that the way to recover during bereavement is to work through the loss, by recognizing, acknowledging, and resolving unconscious and subconscious feelings of attachment and loss through a process of catharsis. M. S. Stroebe (1992/1993) criticized the idea that grief work is a necessary part of recovery. She pointed out that extant definitions of grief work were problematic and that the little empirical work done inside this framework had not yielded consistent results to substantiate this theoretical perspective. Stroebe also contended that the idea of grief work was specific to Western culture and did not hold up cross-culturally.

Along with the psychoanalytic theories came the psychological stress theories, such as the one offered originally by Lazarus and Folkman (1984.) Although this framework was very popular in academia, Lieberman (1992) offered a very useful critique of this approach when it is applied to elderly people. He noted empirical findings that elderly people often do not behave the way stress models would predict during widowhood. Some elderly persons experienced growth in response to the loss, and sometimes a lack of mourning was associated with excellent adaptation. Lieberman concluded that the stress theory may be useful in some circumstances but was limited when applied to elderly persons experiencing bereavement. He also noted that widows appeared to face major tasks in reestablishing and maintaining support and social networks that were not predicted by psychological stress theory.

While we have the same reservations with the grief work hypothesis that Stroebe did, we have concluded that the idea of tasks associated with bereavement has considerable promise in understanding the bereavement of elderly people and in designing interventions. The notion of tasks that must be completed to put a social life back together after a loss is more concrete, focused, and accessible to practitioners and researchers than unconscious and subconscious feelings of attachment and loss.

Our empirical work in bereavement has led us to believe that the bereaved are faced with three tasks to complete before they can put their lives back together after a loss (Steeves, 1996; Steeves & Kahn, 1995; Steeves, Kahn, Wise, & Baldwin, 1993; Steeves, Kahn, Wise, Sepples, & King, 1997). We have used the data from two studies (1-R15-NR02482 & 1-R01-NR03517) to develop and validate this theory. Although the sample from the first study was not exclusively elderly persons, the mean age of the informants was 58 years. In the second study the informants were all elderly persons who had lost a spouse.

Our theory of the tasks of bereavement is based on the notion that death of a loved one challenges the meaning of life for a person. That is, people do not live their lives unmediated as straight experiences. They live them through some sort of framework that gives life meaning. In most cases, this framework is a narrative. In other words, life is a story that we tell to ourselves about who we are and what our lives are about. If we have a normal amount of self-esteem, we are the heroes or heroines of our stories about ourselves and the actions and events in our lives fit together to form an ongoing understandable narrative. It is through this narrative that we establish our social place and define our relationships with others. When a significant character in the narrative of our life dies, the entire narrative meaning may be called into question. The story has suddenly changed and a new direction of the narrative must be established. This seems to be true even when the death is expected, such as for those in a hospice program (the source of our samples). For example, the elderly person may change from being the caregiver of a chronically ill person to being a widow or widower.

The process of establishing this new narrative or new direction, for the ongoing narrative involves three tasks.

1. The first task is the need to complete that section or chapter of the narrative that included the dead person. This is generally done by retelling this narrative over and over. First the retelling is only of the death itself and the events leading up to the death. It is as though the widow or widower is looking at these events for a clue as to how to understand why this chapter of the story ended as it did and where the narrative will go from here. Eventually, the retelling will include the whole relationship with the deceased, from the first meeting until the death. This retelling of the story does not make the pain go away, but the retelling eventually creates a sense of meaning and completeness to that part of the narrative.

2. The second task is to reorder the narrative so that the social fabric of the life of the widow or widower is reknit. Empty roles have to be filled. Some of the widows in our research needed to find a way to have the yard work done and the gutters cleared in the fall. Some widowers needed to learn to cook and keep the checkbook. Both widows and widowers looked for new sources of affection and support. The social relationships that constituted the narrative of their lives had to be realigned so that the place occupied by the dead loved one would not be completely empty.

3. The third task was for these widow or widowers to find a new place for the dead person in the ongoing narrative of their lives. In our research we found that those people who believed in ghosts or believed in the meaningfulness of dreams and could remember their dreams accomplished this third task much more easily than those who did not. It appeared to be easier to negotiate a new social position in a face-to-face encounter. Dead husbands sometimes took on the role of advisers. Widows would say, "When I have a problem, I just try to imagine what he would do in this circumstance." Dead wives sometimes were comforters. Widowers would establish shrines in their houses, with personal objects and photographs of

their wives arranged on a bureau top, for instance, and would go there for comfort. The roles taken on by the newly dead in the narratives of the widow or widower were as complex and as varied as the roles they had held before death.

Do elderly widows or widowers need help in the process of reforming their narratives after the death? If so, how can this be accomplished? We will soon be piloting a project in which hospice volunteers will be used to elicit narratives from the recently bereaved. The volunteers will be trained in the techniques we, as qualitative researchers, used to gather the narratives of our study informants. Our hypothesis is that, since narratives are created to be told, those bereaved elderly persons who have someone who is ready and willing to listen to their multiple tellings of their story will have an easier time accomplishing the three tasks of bereavement than those who do not have a ready listener. Therefore, we will divide the sample into a control group and an intervention group. The control group will have the standard care provided by the hospice we will use to accrue our sample. This includes support telephone calls, the opportunity to join a self-help group, and referral for individual therapy as needed. The intervention group will be visited by volunteers who are trained to listen and elicit stories such as a researcher skilled in qualitative methods. The volunteers will visit on a schedule of decreasing frequency from the week of the funeral for the next 9 months.

Outcome measures for the study will be both qualitative and quantitative. The visits by the volunteers will be tape recorded to see if the bereaved people worked on the tasks of bereavement when given the opportunity to talk. At 9 months after the death, the control group also will be interviewed to determine if they found their own way to work on the tasks of bereavement. The qualitative interviews will be used not only to determine if the tasks of bereavement are being addressed, they will also be used to determine how well the informants believe they are doing in the face of bereavement.

The quantitative measurement of grief is multifaceted, complex, and fraught with empirical and theoretical difficulties, as was demonstrated in the previous discussion. Thus we are still planning and pilot testing possible quantitative instruments. Hansson, Carpenter, and Fairchild (1993), in an interesting review of the measurements that have been used, pointed out the major areas that should be assessed, and their insights will guide our decisions in this area. First, the psychological aspect of grief should be measured, including sadness, depression, rumination, and the like. Second, functioning should be assessed, including role fulfillment, ADL, and lone-liness. Hansson et al. pointed out that there are a number of instruments, many with acceptable psychometrics, that can measure these variables.

Our proposed study certainly will not resolve all the controversies and clear up the confusions in bereavement research. However, we are hoping it will determine the usefulness of viewing bereavement as a challenge to meaning and that meaning can be reestablished through the use of narratives.

SUMMARY AND IMPLICATIONS

This chapter reviewed what has been learned about grief and bereavement in elderly persons. Issues regarding the harmfulness of bereavement and variables affecting responses to grief in elderly persons were explored. The early state of intervention research was noted, and framework for a still-to-be-tested intervention was described.

A few conclusions can be stated at this time. First, as is apparent in the review of the literature, the state of knowledge about bereavement in general and in elderly persons in particular remains tentative. The literature remains equivocal or open to multiple and various interpretations. Probably the most conclusive and reasonable statement that can be made based on the literature is that bereavement is sad and terribly disruptive to life, but most people survive intact. Because of this, it is important that nursing theory and research approach bereavement as a life transition and not as a pathological condition a priori.

Second, the issue of identifying who is most at risk for serious problems in handling grief is a difficult one. At this point, preexisting emotional and social problems seem to be the only reliable predictors of serious difficulties in bereavement. More research clearly is needed. Studies that use the case-control method employed by epidemiologists to determine factors associated with disease would be useful. In such studies, cases, defined as elderly persons experiencing serious problems in bereavement, would be paired with bereaved elderly persons who are not experiencing such problems. Then, differences between the two groups on a range of variables can be investigated retrospectively. As Hahn (1995) noted, this design is useful not only in quantitative studies (which characterize most work in epidemiology), but also can be useful in qualitative studies, using in-depth interviews to compare two groups of similar people who have different outcomes.

Finally, interventions aimed at helping the bereaved so far have only pointed out how complex and not fully understood grieving is. There is no standard of care, or any basis for stating such a standard at this point. Again, more research is needed.

Implications from our discussion follow from the conclusions stated previously. In nursing practice, while it is important to identify persons at risk for complicated grief or problems in bereavement, preexisting problems remain the only good predictor for now. The practitioner should understand that in most cases, elderly persons know what they need to do. Ask them and follow their lead. They may not be able to put what they need to do into words, but they will find a way to work on what they need to do. Just be available for them. A practitioner cannot direct them through the process, because we don't know enough about it to be directive.

A similar implication is for education: novice practitioners, especially students, want protocols. Beyond identifying some of the at-risk people, protocols are not possible. Students need to be taught to listen to the bereaved elderly persons and take their cue from what they hear.

Finally, a policy implication is apparent in the need for more research. Because a phenomenon like grief is complex, multifaceted, and very personal does not mean we cannot come to understand it. Studies that allow us to discover how differences in older adults and in care of bereaved elders contribute to differences in bereavement outcomes are needed now.

REFERENCES

Aber, C. S. (1992). Spousal death, a threat to women's health: Paid work as a "resistance resource." *Image, 24*, 95–99.

Bennett, M. A. (1996). A longitudinal study of well-being in widowed women. *International Journal of Geriatric Psychiatry. 11*, 1005–1010.

Bowlby, J. (1980). *Attachment and loss*. London: Hogarth Press.

Bowling, A. (1988/1989). Who dies after widowhood? A discriminate analysis. *Omega, 19* (2), 135–153.

Brouke, M. P. (1984). The continuum of pre- and post-bereavement grieving. *British Journal of Medical Psychology, 57*, 121–125.

Byrne, G. J. A., & Raphael, B. (1997). The psychological symptoms of conjugal bereavement in elderly men over the first 13 months. *International Journal of Geriatric Psychiatry, 12*, 241–251.

Caserta, M. S., & Lund, D. A. (1993). Intrapersonal resources and the effectiveness of self-help groups for bereaved older adults. *The Gerontologist, 33*, 619–629.

Chenell, S. L, & Murphy, S. A. (1992). Beliefs of the preventability of death among disaster bereaved. *Western Journal of Nursing Research, 14*, 576–594.

Costa, P. T., Zonderman, A. B., & McCrae, R. R. (1991). Personality, defense, coping, and adaptation in older adulthood. In E. M. Cummings, A. L. Greene, & K. Karraker (Eds.), *Life-span developmental psychology: Perspectives on stress and coping* (pp. 277–293). Hillsdale, NJ: Lawrence Erlbaum Associates.

Freud, S. (1917). *Mourning and melancholy*. In J. Strachey (Ed. & Trans.), *Standard edition of the complete works of Sigmund Freud*. London: Hogarth Press.

Glaser, B., & Strauss, A. (1965). *Awareness of dying*. Chicago: Aldine.

Hahn, R. A. (1995). Anthropology and epidemiology: One logic or two? In R. A. Hahn, *Sickness and health* (pp. 99–130). New Haven, CT: Yale University Press.

Hansson, R. O., Carpenter, B. N., & Fairchild, S. K. (1993). Measurement issues in bereavement. In M. S. Strobe, W. Strobe, & R. O. Hansson (Eds.), *Handbook of bereavement: Theory, research, and intervention* (pp. 62–74). New York: Cambridge University Press.

Hays, J., Kasl, S., & Jacobs, S. (1994). Past personal history of dysphoria, social support, and psychological distress following conjugal bereavement. *Journal of the American Geriatrics Society, 42*, 712–718.

Herth, K. (1990). Relationship of hope, coping styles, concurrent losses, and setting to grief resolution in the elderly widow(er). *Research in Nursing and Health, 13*, 109–117

Irwin, M., & Pike, J. (1993). Bereavement, depressive symptoms, and immune function. In M. S. Strobe, W. Strobe, & R. O. Hansson (Eds.), *Handbook of bereavement: Theory, research, and intervention* (pp. 160–174). New York: Cambridge University Press.

Jacobs, S. C. (1987). Psycho-endocrine aspects of bereavement. In S. Zisook (Ed.), *Biopsychosocial aspects of bereavement*. Washington, DC: American Psychological Association.

Kramer, D. (1997). How women relate to terminally ill husbands and their subsequent adjustment to bereavement. *Omega, 34*, 93–106.

Lazarus, R. S., & Folkman, S. (1984). *Stress appraisal and coping*. New York: Springer.

Leahy, J. M. (1992/1993). Depression in women bereaved of a spouse, child or parents. *Omega, 13*, 227–241.

Lehman, D., Ellard, J., & Myrick, R. (1986). Social support for the bereaved: Recipients' and providers' perspectives on what is helpful. *Journal of Consulting and Clinical Psychology, 54*, 438–446.

Lehmand, K., Wortman, D. B., & Williams, A. F. (1987). Long-term effects of losing a spouse or child in a motor vehicle crash. *Journal of Personality and Social Psychology, 52*, 218–231.

Lieberman, M. A. (1992). Limitations of psychological stress models: Studies of widowhood. In M. L. Wykle, E. Kahana, & J. Kowal (Eds.), *Stress and health among the elderly* (pp. 133–150). New York: Springer.

Lieberman, M. A. (1993). Bereavement self-help groups: A review of conceptual and methodological issues. In M. S. Strobe, W. Strobe, & R. O. Hansson (Eds.), *Handbook of bereavement: Theory, research, and intervention* (pp. 411–426). New York: Cambridge University Press.

Lindemann, E. (1944). Symptomatology and management of acute grief. *American Journal of Psychiatry, 101*, 141–148.

Lopata, H. Z. (1993). The support systems of American urban widows. In M. S. Strobe, W. Strobe, & R. O. Hansson (Eds.), *Handbook of bereavement: Theory, research, and intervention* (pp. 381–396). New York: Cambridge University Press.

Lund, D. A., Caserta, M., & Dimond, M. (1993). The course of spousal bereavement in later life. In M. S. Strobe, W. Strobe, & R. O. Hansson (Eds.), *Handbook of bereavement: Theory, research, and intervention* (pp. 240–254). New York: Cambridge University Press.

Matthews, A. M. (1991). *Widowhood in later life*. Toronto: Butterworths.

McKibbin, C. L. (1997). Locus of control perceptions among conjugally bereaved older adults: A pilot study. *International Journal of Aging and Human Development, 44*, 37–45.

Murrell, S. A., Himmelfarb, S., & Phifer, J. F. (1995). Effects of bereavement/loss and pre-event status on subsequent physical health in older adults. In J. Henricks (Ed.), *Health and health care utilization in later life* (pp. 159–177). Amityville, NY: Baywood Press.

Parkes, C. M. (1964a). The effects of bereavement on physical and mental health: A study of widows. *British Medical Journal, 2*, 274–279.

Parkes, C. M. (1964b). Recent bereavement as a cause of mental illness. *British Journal of Psychiatry, 110*, 198–204.

Parkes, C. M. (1965). Bereavement and mental illness. *British Journal of Medical Psychology, 38*, 388–397.

Parkes, C. M. (1971). The first year of bereavement: A longitudinal study of the reaction of London widows to the death of their husbands. *Psychiatry, 33*, 444–466.

Parkes, C. M. (1975/1976). Determinants of outcome following bereavement. *Omega, 6*, 303–323.

Parkes, C. M. (1992). Bereavement and mental health in the elderly. *Reviews in Clinical Gerontology (UK), 2*, 45–51.

Parkes, C. M., & Weiss, R. S. (1983). *Recovery from bereavement*. New York: Basic Books.

Pasternak, R. E., Prigerson, H., Hall, M., Miller, M. D., Fasicska, A., Mazumdar, S., & Reynolds, C. F. (1994). The symptom profile and two-year course of subsyndromal depression in spousally bereaved elders. *American Journal of*

Geriatric Psychiatry, 2, 210–219.

Prigerson, H. G. (1993). Protective psychosocial factors in depression among spousally bereaved elders. *American Journal of Geriatric Psychiatry, 1,* 296–309.

Range, L. M., & Niss, N. M. (1990). Long-term bereavement from suicide, homicide, accidents, and natural deaths. *Death Studies, 14,* 423–433.

Range, L. M., & Thompson, K. (1987). Community responses following suicide, homicide and other deaths: The perspectives of potential comforters. *Journal of Psychology, 12,* 193–198.

Raphael, B., Middleton, W., Martinek, & Misso, V. (1993). Counseling and therapy of the bereaved. In M. S. Strobe, W. Strobe, & R. O. Hansson (Eds.), *Handbook of bereavement: Theory, research, and intervention* (pp. 427–456). New York: Cambridge University Press.

Raphael, B., & Nunn, K. (1988). Counseling the bereaved. *Journal of Social Issues, 44,* 191–206.

Reynolds, C. F., Hoch, C. C., Buysse, D. J., Houck, P. R., Schlernitzaur, M., Pasternak, R. E., Frank, E., Mazumdar, S., & Kupfer, D. J. (1993). Sleep after spousal bereavement: A study of recovery from stress. *Biological Psychiatry, 34,* 791–797.

Rogers, R. G. (1995). Marriage, sex, and mortality. *Journal of Marriage and the Family, 57,* 516–526.

Rosenblatt, P. G. (1993). Grief: The social context of private feelings. In M. S. Strobe, W. Strobe, & R. O. Hansson (Eds.), *Handbook of bereavement: Theory, research, and intervention* (pp. 102–111). New York: Cambridge University Press.

Sanders, C. M. (1979/1980). A comparison of adult bereavement in the death of a spouse, child and parent. *Omega, 10,* 303–322.

Steeves, R. H. (1996). Grief, loss, and the search for meaning. *Oncology Nursing Forum, 23*(6), 897–903.

Steeves, R. H., & Kahn, D. L. (1995). Family perspectives: The tasks of bereavement. *Quality of Life—A Nursing Challenge, 3*(3), 48–55.

Steeves, R. H., Kahn, D. L., Wise, C. T., Sepples, S. B., & King, M. G. (1997). Loss and bereavement: A man's perspective. *Quality of Life: A Nursing Challenge, 5*(1).

Steeves, R. H., Kahn, D. L., Wise, C. T., & Baldwin, A. (1993). The tasks of bereavement for burn center staffs. *Journal of Burn Care and Rehabilitation, 14*(3), 386–397.

Stern, E. M. (1990). *Psychotherapy and the widowed patient.* Binghamton, NY: Haworth Press.

Stroebe, M. S. (1992/1993). Coping with bereavement: A review of the grief work hypothesis. *Omega, 26*(1), 19–42.

Stroebe, M. S., Stroebe, W., & Hansson, R. O. (Eds.). (1993). *Handbook of bereave-*

ment: Theory, research, and intervention. New York: Cambridge University Press.

Ulmer, A., Range, L. M., & Smith, P. C. (1991). Purpose of life: A moderator of recovery from bereavement. *Omega, 23*(4), 279–289.

Van den Hoonaard, D. K. (1994). Paradise lost: Widowhood in a Florida retirement community. *Journal of Aging Studies, 8,* 121–132.

Willert, M. G., Beckwith, B. E., Holm, J. E., & Beckwith, S. K. (1995). A preliminary study of the impact of terminal illness on spouses' social support and coping strategies. *Hospice Journal 10*(4), 35–48.

Zick, C. D., & Smith, K. R. (1991). Patterns of economic change surrounding the death of a spouse. *Journal of Gerontology: Social Sciences, 46,* S310–S320.

Zisook, S., & Shuchter, S. R. (1993). Major depression associated with widowhood. *American Journal of Geriatric Psychiatry, 1,* 316–326.

CHAPTER 6

Grandparents in the Contemporary Family: The Impact of Adult Children's Divorces and Surrogate Parenting

Colleen L. Johnson and Barbara M. Barer

T he 1980s witnessed a rising interest in grandparenting after years of neglect by family researchers. Such interests arose most likely because of increased life expectancy and the potential for more prolonged grandparent-grandchild relationships. For example, *Grandparenthood*, a book edited by Bengtson and Robertson in 1985 captured this surging interest. Two themes were emphasized: the heterogeneity in grandparenting styles and the symbolic functions of the grandparent role. In other words, grandparents were seen as "being there," as sentimentalized or ritualized figures or as "family watchdogs."

By the mid-1990s, the interest in grandparenthood has continued to mount, but the focus has diverged to more urgent issues, namely, that grandparents are potential surrogate parents who can save their grandchildren not only from the effects of parents' divorce, but also from the destructive forces operating in today's society. Evidence of current interest in this subject is found everywhere. The subject dominates programs at national meetings, drawing practitioners in family studies and gerontology.

Recent advice-giving books on grandparenting have taken a more serious turn, moving from tips on how to entertain and babysit grandchildren to how to become parents again (de Toledo & Brown, 1995; Kornhaber & Woodward, 1981). The National Institute on Aging has published not only a public announcement urging research proposals on grandparenting, but also a brochure containing practical information for grandparents raising grandchildren (see Brookdale Newsletters, 1994–1996). There are survival guides for raising a second family and guides to grandparents on how to secure needed services for their grandchildren.

In the process of responding to social change, some gerontologists include the grandparent role as a part of the problem-oriented sense of crisis that drives much of the overall research agenda in gerontology (Myers, 1996; Robertson & Johnson, 1997). While not questioning the urgency of the problems of at-risk children, in this chapter we will first sort out what we know about today's grandparents and how they respond to and are affected by broader social changes now affecting the contemporary family. We will address these issues with a review of the empirical literature about the grandparent role and how it becomes modified with marital changes of adult children.

This chapter reviews the structure and functioning of the family during the divorce process. Where available, the empirical findings from the scant research on grandparents in ethnic families will be included. We also will analyze how grandparents define their roles when faced with a child's divorce. Finally, we will review the policy issues related to grandparents who are functioning as surrogate parents. Our experiences with this topic come from two research endeavors: a 5-year study of grandparenting in divorcing families in Northern California suburbs and studies of inner-city families of older Blacks.

FAMILY REORGANIZATION WITH DIVORCE AND REMARRIAGE

Marital instability is more common today than at any time in our history, perhaps reflecting a widespread rejection of the norms of the conventional nuclear family (Poponoe, 1993). The number of divorces have quadrupled since 1960, and it is estimated that as many as two thirds of the recently married people will divorce (Bumpass, 1990). In fact, the one-parent household may become the dominant pattern. Projections suggest that from birth to age 17, 70% of Whites and 94% of Blacks will live at some point in a one-parent household (Hofferth, 1985). These high rates come not only from divorce but also from the increased number of new mothers who do not marry (24% of the Whites and 62% of the Blacks) (Preston, 1984).

Longino and Earle (1996) outline the major demographic trends that affect grandparenting. The high divorce rate along with the increased number of single-parent households in the baby boom generation have increased the size of the low-income population. At the same time, with women's entrance into the major professions, two-career marriages create more upper income households, resulting in a two-tier system of stratification. Moreover, with later marriage, later childbearing, and fewer children born, a wider age gap exists between generations. Thus the period of grandparenting increasingly occurs with older grandparents, not only from this altered age structure, but also from the greater longevity of grandparents.

It has been estimated that approximately 14.1 million older Americans spend a mean of 13.7 hours a week providing supportive services to grandchildren. That level represents a full-time annual effort of 4.2 million workers and is valued monetarily at $17.4 to $29.1 billion annually (Bass & Caro, 1996). If fewer grandparents will be available to assist increased numbers of grandchildren, as Presser (1989) maintains, then more social services will be needed in the future.

As a process of reorganization occurs following marital dissolution, these changes have far-reaching effects on the individuals involved and on the organization of the kinship system. Grandparents are particularly affected, for one half of them with ever-married children are estimated to have at least one divorced child (Spitze, Logan, Deane, & Zerger, 1994).

STRUCTURAL EFFECTS ON GRANDPARENTING

Marital Dissolution After Death and Divorce

In the past, the loss of a parent occurred with death, leading to different effects than those after a divorce. For example, divorce is not recognized with rituals and institutional mechanisms such as those following a death that lessen the effects of loss and mobilize supports to the bereaved (Lopata, 1973). In fact, divorced individuals have more difficulty meeting their kinship obligations than the stably married (Rossi & Rossi, 1990). Those individuals who are experiencing marital changes enter a period of social limbo where norms are vague about how to respond. In other words, society permits divorce but has not provided for its consequences (Goode, 1956). Also unlike death, divorce and remarriage are more complicated processes, because they do not replace the loss of a parent; instead, these marital changes rearrange existing personnel (Furstenberg & Spanier, 1984).

Economic Strains

In the process of reallocating existing financial resources, the needs of two households must be met. Consequently, far greater costs are entailed in the formation of new households (Matthews & Sprey, 1984). According to some views, in fact, children's problems after parents divorce may be traced mostly to the shortage of money (Longfellow, 1979). Economic problems are insidious after divorce, particularly for women (Longino & Earle, 1996). Their economic status worsens after a divorce, while divorced men generally have improved economic resources (Wallerstein & Kelly, 1979; Weitzman, 1985). Given the economic strains created by marital changes, it is understandable that divorcing parents are likely to turn to their own parents for help. Thus there also are economic repercussions for grandparents, many of whom work. If they must take on a parenting role, their economic resources will be affected (Simon-Rusinowitz, Krach, Marks, Piktialis, & Wilson, 1996).

Norms of Noninterference and Grandchildren's Needs

With the norm of privacy that governs relationships between nuclear households (Laslett, 1978), grandparents had usually avoided interfering in their childrens' lives. They had been intimate but at a distance from their children and grandchildren. As a child's marriage is dissolving, however, family activities usually become more public in the midst of conflict, and in some cases, substance abuse, new sexual liaisons, and developmental problems of grandchildren. While respecting the norm of noninterference in their child's family, grandparents are uncertain as to how they can intervene in the interests of their grandchildren. If they do intervene, they cross that boundary of privacy, and, in the process, they may learn more about their child's life than they want to know (Johnson, 1988b).

The Lineage Connection

The custody arrangements following divorce are the most important determinants of the actions of grandparents. As occupants of a derived role, the grandparent-grandchild relationship is mediated by the parents. With custody usually granted to women, maternal grandparents usually have no difficulties gaining access to their grandchildren (Furstenberg & Spanier, 1984; Johnson, 1989). Paternal grandparents, however, may have to mediate with a former daughter-in-law if their own son cannot provide them with access. While she may no longer be a son's wife, she is usually still viewed as the mother of their grandchildren. Some grandparents also may want to compensate for a son's deficiencies as a parent. Thus they do not want to sever their relationship with a former child-in-law. Any coalition with his former wife, however, may create tension with their son, and, understandably, it competes with their allegiance to a son's new wife in the event he remarries.

Remarriage

Remarriage of a child or former child-in-law further complicates an already vague and confusing period of family change as new families are formed. Grandparents must navigate through an expanded kinship system that has few rules or expectations (Cherlin, 1978; Johnson, 1989). If they are to continue a close relationship with grandchildren, they potentially accumulate new children-in-law and stepgrandchildren. Where they have difficulty continuing to see their grandchildren when they choose, they may lose them in the midst of the fast-paced changes in the families (Johnson & Barer, 1987).

CULTURAL DIVERSITY IN FAMILY STRUCTURE

Other than the growing literature on Black families, the systematic study of broader cultural diversity in grandparents' roles in ethnic families is in a preliminary stage. While most researchers know intuitively that Asian and Hispanic families differ from non-Hispanic Whites, there is only a sparse literature on just how they differ. Beyond the members of nuclear families, very little is known about grandparents' status during the process of kinship reorganization with marital change, and virtually nothing is known on how they respond to a child's divorce. We do know that Black children are more likely to live with a grandparent: 12.3% do in comparison to 3.7% White and 5.6% Hispanic. Nevertheless, the incidence of White grandchildren living with grandparents has increased 54% since 1980 in comparison to a 24% increase for Blacks and a 40% increase for Hispanics (Saluter, 1992).

For operational purposes, three models of the family provide a convenient classification to capture the diversity in ethnic families and to predict how grandparents may react to the divorce of a child (Johnson, 1995). First, *the traditional family* model has a hierarchical family structure with the old dominant over the young and males over women. Such families stress respect for elders, strong obligations to family interests over personal interests, and interdependence (Cowgill & Holmes, 1972; Johnson, 1977, 1985b). Strong filial norms undoubtedly enhance the status of grandparents. Evidence suggests that helping networks are stronger in the traditional family (Cantor & Little, 1985; Weeks & Cuellar, 1981). Where marital instability occurs, the interdependence among multiple family members would ease the strains of caring for grandchildren. It is likely that other relatives would assist a grandparent in his or her activities with grandchildren.

Typical of this family model are Asian families with their Confucian principles that extol an age hierarchy, one that stands in marked contrast to American values (Johnson, 1977). Hispanic groups and some European Catholic groups also typify such patterns of interdependence among an extended family group, but because they are not monolithic groups, it is difficult to generalize (Johnson, 1985b; Markides & Mindel, 1987). The number of minority and ethnic older people are increasing more rapidly than the non-Hispanic White population (Treas, 1995), and in most groups, the grandparent role tends to be more important than in the dominant group in the United States. Consequently, ethnic grandparents living in ethnic enclaves are likely to play authoritative roles (Longino & Earle, 1996). However, since traditional family values are often incongruent with the dominant American pattern, these families may be affected by assimilation and intermarriage of their younger generations.

Second, in contrast to the traditional family model, the much criticized Parsonian *nuclear model* has until recently dominated our thinking about the family (Parsons, 1965). This domestic group consists of parents and dependent children. It has two functions: the socialization of children and the stabilization of the adult personality. In its ideal form, this family type has been criticized as a stereotype for White middle-class families, but one that many see as unachievable or undesirable. Since divorced individuals are more likely to remarry than are widowed individuals, divorce does not necessarily end such a form. In fact, the high incidence of remarriages has been identified as "serial monogamy." This family type is relatively egalitarian in comparison to traditional families, with its values giving priorities to independence and individual interests over family interests. The egalitarian family is residentially and emotionally separate from its kinship group, and many of its functions have been transferred to outside institutions.

With the rising divorce rate, this family type is more vulnerable, because the household has been based on the marriage of the parents (Bohannon, 1971). Members of such families have usually maintained some distance from relatives, and their values on independence discourage close connections beyond the nuclear unit. Understandably, older family members also are vulnerable, because they experience the isolating effects of having a household separate from children. They also may be emotionally and socially distant from their grandchildren. Despite its deficiencies, most observers conclude that this family is the goal, not only of the White majority, but also of those undergoing assimilation or upward mobility.

Third, *the opportune family* is used here to identify some alternatives to the nuclear family when problems such as divorce, poverty, sexual preferences, or death lead to diminished family resources. This family type has flexible definitions about who is family and for whom one has responsibility (Johnson, 1988c). From the grandparents' perspective, their definition of how they are related to a former child-in-law is usually revised. Responses often are driven by the needs of a given situation even when distinguishing who is part of one's own family. For example, relationships can be based on bonds of affection rather than blood or marriage. Sometimes the kinship group following marital changes are labeled "divorce and remarried chains" (Furstenberg, 1981). This form of family was found among one third of the White families in our study who were going through a divorce (Johnson, 1988c). Relationships in these kinship networks can be friendly but at a distance or, in contrast, be active helping networks.

Families with flexible boundaries are commonly found among Blacks, where a communal philosophy about family is the norm. The practice of raising the children of others has been a long tradition in Black families, so children in dissolving families are usually incorporated into other households. In fact, Black children are more likely than White children to live in extended family households (Ruggles, 1994). Roles are flexible and interchangeable, and the family has the capacity to absorb foster children (Aschenbrenner, 1973; Johnson & Barer, 1990). Consequently, in its ideal form at least, the household structures may include several adults. The grandmother in Black families occupies an esteemed role, and she makes practical contributions to the family. She also is an important authority figure (Cherlin & Furstenberg, 1986).

THE ATTRIBUTES OF THE GRANDPARENT ROLE

Divorce and grandparenting converge upon two socially ambiguous phenomena. Given the disruptive effects of divorce and the conflicts during the processes of family reorganization, grandparents are placed in a nebulous position. Unlike parenting, with its explicit and legally enforced norms of responsibility, expectations for grandparenting are only vaguely specified. The divorce has created needs which grandparents are the most logical relation to meet, but the White, mostly middle-class grandparents in our study had difficulty making decisions about how to proceed. Because the parents of the grandchildren mediate their actions, grandparents are not free agents. In interviews with grandmothers shortly after their children divorced, we asked them what they felt they should do. In analyzing their responses, we found both prescriptions and proscriptions—the shoulds and should nots of grandparenting (Johnson, 1983):

Prescriptions:	Proscriptions:
1. Be there	Don't interfere
2. Be an advocate	Don't be judgmental
3. Provide family continuity	Don't give advice
4. Be loving	Don't buy love
5. Be a liaison with parents	Don't discipline
6. Be a source of security	Don't be a fuddy-duddy
7. Make it easier for parents	Don't expect too much
8. Babysit	Don't nag
9. Just enjoy them	Don't be dull
10. Be fun to be with	Don't be old-fashioned

In their prescriptions of the role, they preferred that grandparents simply be there to help when needed, yet they also should have some symbolic functions as a stabilizing family force and a symbol of family continuity. The "should nots" brought forth more lengthy discussions about the one-way flow of benefits in their role. Although they should babysit, they should not discipline grandchildren, give advice, be too protective, or judgmental. Most of these "should nots" imply that they should not transmit their own values. They cannot be dull or old-fashioned, for that would imply they are not fun figures. Most important, the proscriptive norms are more explicit than most of the prescriptive norms. "Being there" or providing family continuity or self-esteem are vague, but such actions as interfering or nagging or even being dull are more clearly communicated.

Dilemmas About Grandparenting

Uncertainties about the role of grandparents may become accentuated during the divorce process because of other qualities of the grandparent role. Earlier researchers on grandparenting tended to depict the role in terms of style—"the funseeker," "the formal," "the distant," or "the parent surrogate" grandmother (Neugarten & Weinstein, 1964; Robertson, 1977). Moreover, life satisfaction is not associated with the grandparenting role (Wood & Robertson, 1976), and, in return, grandchildren are not usually providers of support for older people (Johnson, 1985a). In fact, a common saying among grandparents is, "When in need, one good friend is more important than a dozen grandchildren" (Blau, 1973). The role has been described as having a ritualized quality and is often considered a "state of mind" rather than a functioning role (Kahana & Kahana, 1970). These more ethereal qualities result from the fact that most grandparents reject the authority and nurturing functions of parenting. The grandmothers in our study also echoed the preferences of one, "I never want to be the parent—I just want to enjoy my grandchildren."

When presented with the divorce of an offspring and the opportunity to substitute for parents in meeting the basic needs of the grandchildren, the grandmothers in our study were somewhat confused about their potential functions. They tended to define their role in accordance with the situation and then determined the level of their involvement situationally, depending on the needs of their children, grandchildren, and even children-in-law. Most grandmothers do not want to be disciplinarians, for their style then rests not only on the satisfaction of their grandchildren's needs for pleasure but also those of their own. As modern grandmothers, they reject the traditional aspects of the role, the one portraying a nurturing, domestic woman who slaves all day over a hot stove. Instead, they emphasize the playful aspects of the role: a grandmother should be fun to be with, not a meddlesome, controlling woman (Johnson, 1983, 1985a).

Given these characteristics, the role is one of diversity rather than a central tendency (Troll, 1980, 1983). As children divorce and the needs of grandchildren mount, the qualities of the role are likely to change. Sometimes grandparents are the only ones who can help financially or with hands-on care. Nevertheless, grandparents in these situations are uncertain about their course of action. They cannot step in uninvited or against the wishes of a child or former child-in-law, so they must personally negotiate with them about what is expected of them. In other words, they do not generally see themselves as free agents. Any actions they take are potentially constrained by the parents of their grandchildren, only one of whom is related after a divorce (Johnson, 1983, 1985a, 1988a).

Given the high needs of their children and grandchildren, the major dilemma facing these grandmothers when a child divorces was commonly expressed with ambivalence, "If I do too much for my grandchildren, I will have to do it all. If I do too little, I might lose them." This response reflects the quandary created by the voluntary character of the role in a situation where needs are high. If the situation demands that they take over some parenting functions, grandmothers feel that they risk becoming overburdened. Obviously, the possibility of being a surrogate parent was not on the agenda of most grandmothers. Since there were only vague and often implicit expectations for the role, grandmothers in general were hesitant to take over responsibilities that were not clearly defined. Explanations often entailed a rationalization that the parent role should not be repeated, "I have paid my dues. It is time for me to think of myself." Consequently, after a child's divorce, grandparents describe their ad hoc responses, "I just roll with the punches."

GRANDPARENTS' ACTIONS

While the empirical and clinical research literature on divorce is prolific as is an increasingly informative literature on grandparenting (Kivett, 1991), only a few studies have combined research on a grandparent's role during a child's divorce process (Gladstone, 1988; Johnson, 1983, 1985a, 1988b, 1988a, 1988c; Johnson & Barer, 1987; Matthews & Sprey, 1984; Spitze et al., 1994; Sprey & Matthews, 1982). Despite some ambivalence and uncertainty among grandparents, our research found that most rose to the occasion and extended assistance to their divorcing children and their children. Three quarters had at least weekly contact with their children (Johnson, 1983, 1988a, 1988b; Johnson & Barer, 1987). Although these women tended to have less contact with their grandchildren than with their children, most extended considerable assistance to both generations in the period immediately following the divorce. More than two thirds provided financial help and most provided some services at least intermittently. Nevertheless, there was considerable variation in their level of activity. Over 40 months, there was some decline in their involvement with grandchildren, but their relationship with their children was less subject to change. Greater changes, however, took place among paternal grandparents, who were likely to experience sharp declines over time in their involvement with grandchildren of divorce.

In our study, most grandparents who had initially taken on parental responsibilities for their grandchildren, no longer did so after 3 years. Their initial response was a stop-gap measure intended to ease the immediate strains in their child's and grandchildren's lives. Thus grandparents with such responsibilities rarely viewed the arrangement as permanent, but rather they looked forward to a time when they were free of such a commitment. If their responsibilities persisted, conflict with their children invariably arose, conflicts accentuated by an involuntary role reversal and often a regression on the child's part.

Grandparenting activities vary after the divorce of a child, not only because of the cultural diversity in this country, but also because their actions stem mostly from immediate needs. Other factors also are involved:

1. Diversity in how the role is performed following a child's divorce can be traced in large part to the grandparent's age. The mean age of grandparents is 45, with a range from approximately 25 to 100 years (Kivett, 1991). The age of grandparents is one of the most frequently cited determinants of the role (Johnson, 1985a, 1988a; Kivett, 1991; Sprey & Matthews, 1982; Thomas, 1986). Younger grandmothers usually have younger grandchildren who need more help after a divorce; consequently, younger grandparents are more active with grandchildren. These variations also stem from the diminishing energy of grandparents with their increasing age and the decreasing needs for help as the grandchildren mature.

2. With a divorce of a child, gender-based kinship positions also are very important. In the absence of divorce, maternal and paternal grand-

parents see grandchildren at about the same frequency. With divorce, however, maternal grandmothers have more contact, while contact decreases with paternal grandmothers (Cherlin & Furstenberg, 1986). Consequently, custody in a large part determines the grandparent role. Maternal grandparents are more active than paternal grandparents because daughters are much more likely to have custody (Sprey & Matthews, 1982).

In general, relationships between generations have a strong matrilateral bias. Bonds among mothers, daughters, and granddaughters are stronger and more enduring than those in the male line (Hagestad, 1990). Spitze et al. (1994) found out that the gender-based kinship position is a significant determinant, with both maternal grandmothers and grandfathers being more important than either paternal grandparents. Divorced daughters have more contact with parents than divorced sons and married daughters, and they receive more aid from them (Johnson, 1988c). On the contrary, married sons receive more babysitting help than divorced sons.

When marriages fail, divorced women are more likely than divorced men to have lower standards of living while men's standards usually improve (Rossi & Rossi, 1990). Women also are responsible for the children, often with no financial or social support from ex-husbands. In fact, a national survey found that a year after divorce, one half the men had no contact with their children (Furstenberg, Nord, Peterson, & Zill, 1983). Consequently, women have a greater developmental stake in maintaining their relationships with parents. Rossi and Rossi also suggest, however, that a woman's return to a more dependent status with her parents is not unilateral, but one of eventual interdependence as her parents later need her help.

3. In both intact and disrupted families, parents in the middle generation usually function as mediators between their parents and their children. Consequently, they influence both the quality and quantity of the interactions between grandparents and grandchildren. If a parent has a close relationship with his or her parent, then the grandchildren will have a closer relationship with their grandparents (Hodgson, 1992; Kennedy, 1992). A national survey found that the quality of intergenerational relationships is influenced by divorce (Umberson, 1992). When either a parent or adult child divorces, intergenerational relationships are substantially more strained, Umberson concludes, most often because of financial problems.

In any case, a child's divorce is usually an upsetting experience to grandparents (E. S. Johnson, 1981), and the additional strains from economic shortages may heighten the strains during that period. More subtle family processes also are undoubtedly affected by divorce. Thompson and Walker (1987) found that grandmothers were most likely to have a global family feeling, where closeness to their daughters and grand-daughters is indistinguishable. Granddaughters, on the contrary, differentiate between their feelings about their mother and grandmother. Such family feelings may be related to older people's tendency to refer to grandchildren and other relatives as a generic category that infers equal feelings for all. Nor do they single out specific characteristics of an individual (Troll, 1994).

In our study, the actual relationships with a divorcing adult child seemed to depend on the history of that relationship (Johnson, 1988b). For example, if an adult child had long had an interdependent role with parents, that relationships was strengthened after a divorce. Other divorcing parents who had always been independent from their parents tended to have a distant relationship; so after their divorce, they still maintained a private family unit. Still others had divorce and remarriage networks that blurred family boundaries between relatives of blood, marriage, and divorce; so grandparents were included along with relatives accumulated by marital changes.

SURROGATE PARENTING
IN AN ERA OF FAMILY CHANGE

The issue of grandparents as surrogate parents is dominated by ideological stances regarding basic definitions of the family. On the one hand, the nuclear family model is condemned for being color-blind, outdated, and impractical in today's world (Stacy, 1993). A normal family with both parents and dependent children, these critics claim, is irrelevant in an era of altered female roles, a high divorce rate, single mothering, unconventional unions, and gay and lesbian families of choice. When the nuclear family is the norm, other family types risk being defined as deviant. Others maintain that the nuclear family is the optimal setting for raising children (Poponoe, 1993). Hence the steep decline in the prevalence of the nuclear family has serious consequences for children. In the face of these family changes, the potentials for grandparental intervention become more important. Recent family critics advocate for a closer affiliation between grandparents and their grandchildren. As previous research indicates, however, for a variety of reasons, most grandparents are hesitant about reassuming a parental role. Instead, at their stage of life, they want to be free from such responsibilities (Robertson & Johnson, 1997).

These compelling concerns come at a time when 5% of dependent children live with a grandparent, a 40% rise in 2 decades (Robertson, 1995). Logically, some of these grandparents are surrogate parents, for a national survey in 1988 found that 2.6% of the children live with a grandparent without a parent present (Solomon & Marx, 1995). Surrogate parenting is needed when the marital breakdown is associated with poverty, substance abuse, and teenage births, all of which undermine the parents' capacity to raise their children. As a consequence, the grandmothers, who are likely to become surrogate parents in such situations, are usually poorer than the norm and may need assistance themselves (Robertson, 1995).

In addressing these issues, three questions arise. (1) Are grandparents as surrogate parents beneficial to grandchildren? (2) Are such arrangements beneficial to grandparents? (3) What policies and social services are needed?

Effects on Grandchildren

Most literature about young children being parented by grandparents comes from clinical research that reports an increase in custodial grandchildren being referred for treatment (Hetherington, 1989; Shore & Hayslip, 1994). These children had most likely experienced some trauma during the period when their parents' marriage was dissolving, so it is impossible to sort out the antecedents of psychological problems, whether it be from the family breakdown or the process of becoming surrogate grandchildren. A recent report offers more sound empirical findings. By using the 1988 National Health Supplement, Solomon and Marx (1995) found that children being raised by their grandparents fared very well in comparison to children in families with only one biological parent (either a single-parent family or a stepfamily). Children raised by their grandparents are healthier and have fewer behavioral problems than those raised in alternate family forms. Black children raised by grandparents do not differ from their White counterparts in their adaptation except in having higher potential problems with teachers.

Effects on Grandparents

The White House Conference on Aging (1995) addressed the difficulties that custodial grandparents are facing. During the conference, it was estimated that two million children are being raised by grandparents, and one half of the grandparent-headed households have incomes of less than $20,000, with 27% having incomes below the poverty level. The usual support services available for dependent children do not generally extend to older people caring for them. This report found that grandparents forced into the role of primary caregiver experience a major upheaval, stress, financial problems, and family conflict.

In one third of the cases studied by Presser (1989), grandparents caring for grandchildren often held outside jobs. They experience sleep deprivation, overwhelming responsibilities, and chronic health problems. Moreover, the grandparents who are still working face the usual difficulties of arranging flexible work schedules and affordable child care (Simon-Rusinowitz et al., 1996). Grandparents with legal responsibility for grandchildren are more adversely affected in their lifestyles than those who provide day care or those who have noncustodial grandchildren in their households (Jendrek, 1993, 1994). More telling is indirect evidence: Larsen (1991), for example, reported that the purpose of 300 support groups for grandparents was to help them deal with the stresses of raising grandchildren and with their resentments about having such responsibilities.

Black Grandmothers

As we noted previously, the responsibilities of surrogate parenting rest heavily on women and minorities. Black grandmothers provide more care for grandchildren than Whites and do so without substitute helpers (White-Means & Thornton, 1990). Black surrogate grandmothers have a positive effect on their grandchildren, who do as well as children in two-parent families (Kellam, Ensminger, & Turner, 1977). Two studies of Black grandmothers caring for the children of their drug-addicted children, however, speak of heavy costs for custodial grandparents. Burton's findings (1992) indicate that the rich helping resources usually associated with Black extended families do not seem to operate in such situations. While these grandmothers found their grandchildren emotionally rewarding, the parenting tasks entailed high physical and psychological stressors. Likewise, Minkler and Roe (1993, 1996) speak of the heavy burden on grandparents: health problems, economic difficulties, lack of public support, social isolation, and the problems of raising high-needs grandchildren.

In family structure, younger Blacks are more likely than Whites to remain in or return to their parents' household (Glick & Lin, 1986). Thus three-generation households are more common among them. Not only are older Blacks more likely than Whites to have grandchildren in the household, they also are more likely to be raising children other than their own (Cherlin & Furstenberg, 1986). The Martins' study (1978) found that some grandmothers felt that their family was taking advantage of their "goodness" by sending them too many children to raise. Burton and Bengtson (1985) also found that selected women were singled out for the maternal role for the children of other family members.

The extent to which the culturally variant structure of Black families is related to familistic values or to economic marginality is uncertain (Dilworth-Anderson, Burton, & Turner, 1993; Gratton, 1987). It appears that some features of the Black family are an outgrowth of slavery and later traditions in the rural South. One feature was the belief that everyone belonged to somebody; so large numbers of children were absorbed into extended families, either their own or those of nonrelatives. The practice of raising the children of others was part of these family values (Staples & Johnson, 1993), and grandparents particularly were important agents of socialization. Later in urban areas, those grandmothers that live with daughters are seen as more active and supportive of children and grandchildren than those who live apart (Gratton, 1987). Nevertheless, Black grandparents, like their White counterparts, prefer to live near but not with their descendants (Jackson, 1986; Wilson, 1986).

Obviously, the current urban setting may find grandparents "under siege" as they must deal with violence and the erratic behavior of drug-addicted children (Burton, 1992). Burton and Dilworth-Anderson (1991) point out that grandmothers with drug-addicted children may be responsible for not just one grandchild but several. With the early age of childbearing, the age of grandmother caregivers can range from the late 20s to advanced old age. Grandmothers in each age group face a varied set of problems.

Policy Issues of Surrogate Parenting

Custodial grandparents face a host of difficulties in finding financial assistance, health insurance, housing, or even in gaining legal rights to make decisions regarding their grandchildren's health care and education (Chalfie, 1994). First, financial problems loom large. Minority grandparents who have custody of grandchildren face even more stressors than Whites because they have lower financial resources to begin with, a problem compounded by the serious risks of crime-ridden urban neighborhoods (Burton, 1992).

Second, their legal rights are minimal. Recent court decisions conclude that issues such as grandparent visitation rights are moral issues lying outside the domain of the law. Consequently, parents cannot be forced by the law to permit visits between their parents or parents-in-law and their children (Wilhite, 1987). Even more illogical are government policies that differentiate between grandparents who are raising their own grandchildren and foster-care parents who are raising unrelated children. In fact, biological grandparents are not even granted the same government benefits received by foster parents, such as financial compensation, psychological counseling, and clothing allowances (Minkler & Roe, 1993).

Third, grandparents acting as surrogate parents have difficulty securing the usual safety-net services such as Aid to Dependent Children, Medicaid, and Food Stamps. The American Association of Retired Persons' Grandparent Information Services has provided tips for grandparents in untangling the web of public programs and learning how to apply for such services.

The White House Conference on Aging (1995) offered the following 10 context resolutions that conceptualize the scope of the needs of custodial grandparents and the policy changes required to address their needs:

1. Grant grandparents legal surrogate decision-making authority.
2. Provide them with culturally and linguistically sensitive information and referral services.
3. Establish comprehensive programs for grandparents that include respite and day care, legal assistance, mental health and advocacy services, health care and substance abuse treatment.
4. Promote the development of caregiver support groups.
5. Provide financial, social, and legal supports as needed.
6. Remove legal and administrative barriers to safety-net programs.
7. Educate human service providers about grandparent caregiver households.
8. Expand the Administration on Aging programs to include grandparent support groups at senior centers.
9. Protect visitation rights of grandparents.
10. Promote intergenerational programs to strengthen the family unit.

CONCLUSIONS

The divorce process entails a process of family reorganization that affects not only members of the dissolving nuclear family but also the grandparents. Unlike family change after the death of a parent, divorce rearranges both personnel and resources into a more complex and often economically strapped family situation. Financial problems, parental distraction, conflict, and demoralization are common. In many cases, grandparents are the only ones available to intervene, but their actions are constrained by the parents of their grandchildren, only one of whom is a relative. Thus maternal grandmothers are most often the supporters, while paternal grandmothers may have difficulty securing access to their grandchildren.

In the literature, the grandparent role is viewed as one of diversity, not only because of the cultural diversity in this country, but also because the role itself is not normatively regulated as to the rights and responsibilities of grandparents. Grandparents occupy a derived role where any actions they take are mediated by the parents of their grandchildren. As a consequence, a consistent theme concerns the ambiguity in the role, perhaps reflecting the common usage of the concept "style" to describe variations in the role. Most grandparents, however, respond to the needs a divorce creates by coming to the immediate aid of their grandchildren. Nevertheless, grandparents reject the pressures to become surrogate parents, and when those responsibilities are forced upon them, they experience considerable stress.

With the high divorce rate in the United States and the sharp increase in one-parent households, more and more members of our population are vulnerable to the predictable consequences, when one parent leaves the household. Given current trends, future projections about the needs of families and older people must take the ripple effects of divorce into account. In such situations, the financial and social resources of families are drastically reduced. The divorce process alters the pattern of reciprocity between generations. Family help in child care is a major need and one that will only increase. Any increase in the divorce rate may come at a point in time when the number and availability of grandparents are decreasing. As more younger people divorce, they might find not only fewer grandparents but also grandparents less available to help them because of their health, competing commitments, or their personal wishes for autonomy from family responsibilities (Presser, 1989). Likewise, divorcing children are usually too distracted to be attentive to their parents. As more older people are affected by divorce, either their own, or their children's, future older people may experience a decline in family supports. Children may not reach a stage in their lives when they can help their parents. Since most supports to older people come from children, consequently, this pattern of support cannot be ensured in the future.

At the same time, entitlement programs are being cut back with the expectations that families will see to the needs of dependent children and older people. With the widespread publicity about grandparents as surrogate parents, some justification may be used to cut further benefits to families. Given the fact that the burdens of surrogate or custodial grandparenting fall mainly on women, the poor, and minorities, the future distribution of public benefits may be critical. It is hoped that future policy makers will be aware of the adverse effects of marital instability, for the ripple effects undermine the situation not only of dependent children, but also of several generations of grandparents.

REFERENCES

Abraham, I., Buckwalter, K., Neese, J., & Fox, J. (1994). Mental health of rural elderly: A research agenda for nursing. *Issues in Mental Health Nursing, 15*(3), 203–213.

Aschenbrenner, J. (1973). Extended families among black Americans. *Journal of Comparative Family Studies, 4,* 257–268.

Bass, S. A., & Caro, F. G. (1996). The economic value of grandparent assistance. *Generations, XX*(1), 29–38.

Bengtson, V. L., & Robertson, J. F. (Eds.). (1985). *Grandparenthood.* Beverly Hills, CA: Sage.

Blau, Z. (1973). *Old age in a changing society.* New York: Viewpoints.

Bohannon, P. (1971). *Divorce and after.* New York: Anchor Books.

Brookdale Newsletter. (1994–1996). *Parenting grandchildren: A voice for grandparents.* Washington, DC: AARP Grandparent Information Center.

Bumpass, L. L. (1990). What's happening to the family? Interactions between demographic and institutional change. *Demography, 27,* 483–498.

Burton, L. (1992). Black grandparents rearing children of drug-addicted parents: Stressors, outcomes, and social service needs. *The Gerontologist, 32,* 744–751.

Burton, L. M., & Bengtson, V. (1985). Black grandmothers: Issues of timing and continuity of roles. In V. Bengtson & J. Robertson (Eds.), *Grandparenthood* (pp. 61–78). Beverly Hills, CA: Sage.

Burton, L., & Dilworth-Anderson, P. (1991). The intergenerational family roles of aged Black Americans. *Marriage and Family Review, 16,* 311–330.

Cantor, M. H., & Little, V. (1985). Aging and social care. In R. Binstock & L. George (Eds.), *Handbook of aging and the social sciences* (pp. 745–781). New York: Van Nostrand Reinhold.

Chalfie, D. (1994). *Going it alone: A closer look at grandparents parenting grandchildren.* Washington, DC: AARP Women's Initiative.

Cherlin, A. (1978). Remarriage as an incomplete institution. *American Journal of Sociology, 84,* 634–650.

Cherlin, A., & Furstenberg, F. (1986). *The new American grandparent: A place in the family, a life apart.* New York: Basic Books.

Cowgill, D. O., & Holmes, L. D. (1972). *Aging and modernization.* New York: Appleton Century-Crofts.

deToledo, S., & Brown, D. E. (1995). *Grandparents as parents: A survival guide for raising a second family.* New York: Guildford Press.

Dilworth-Anderson, P., Burton, L. M., & Turner, W. L. (1993). The importance of values in the study of culturally diverse families. *Family Relations, 42,* 238–242.

Furstenberg, F. (1981). Remarriage and intergenerational relations. In R. Fogel, E. Hatfield, S. Keesler, & E. Shanas (Eds.), *Aging: Stability and change in the family* (pp. 115–142). New York: Academic Press.

Furstenberg, F., Nord, C. W., Peterson, J. L., & Zill, N. (1983). The life course of children of divorce: Marital disruption and parental contact. *American Sociological Review, 48,* 656–668.

Furstenberg F., & Spanier, G. (1984) *Recycling the family: Remarriage after divorce.* Beverly Hills, CA: Sage.

Gladstone, J. W. (1988). Perceived changes in grandmother-grandchild relations following a child's separation or divorce. *The Gerontologist, 28,* 66–72.

Glick, P. C., & Lin, S. (1986). More young adults are living with their parents: Who are they? *Journal of Marriage and the Family, 48*(1), 107–112.

Goode, W. (1956). *Women in divorce.* New York: Free Press.

Gratton, B. (1987). Familism among the Black and Mexican-American elderly: Myth or reality? *Journal of Aging Studies, 1*(1), 19–32.

Hagestad, G. O. (1990). Social perspectives on the life course. In R. Binstock & L. George (Eds.), *Handbook of aging and the social sciences.* New York: Academic Press.

Hetherington, E. M. (1989). Coping with family transitions: Winners, losers, and survivors. *Child Development, 60,* 1–14.

Hodgson, L. G. (1992). Adult grandchildren and their grandparents: The enduring bond. *International Journal of Aging and Human Development, 34,* 209–225.

Hofferth, S. L. (1985). Updating children's life course. *Journal of Marriage and the Family, 47,* 93–115.

Jackson, J. (1986). Black grandparents: Who needs them? In R. Staples (Ed.), *The Black family: Essays and studies* (pp. 186–194). Belmont, CA: Wadsworth.

Jendrek, M. P. (1993). Grandparents who parent their grandchildren: Effects on lifestyle. *Journal of Marriage and the Family, 55,* 609–621.

Jendrek, M. P. (1994). Grandparents who parent their grandchildren: Circumstances and decisions. *The Gerontologist, 34*, 206–216.

Johnson, C. L. (1977). Interdependence, reciprocity and indebtedness: An analysis of Japanese American kinship relations. *Journal of Marriage and the Family, 39*, 351–363.

Johnson, C. L. (1983). A cultural analysis of the grandmother. *Research in Aging, 5*, 547–567.

Johnson, C. L. (1985a). Grandparenting options in divorcing families: An anthropological perspective. In V. Bengston & J. Robertson (Eds.), *Grandparenthood* (pp. 81–96). Beverly Hills, CA: Sage.

Johnson, C. L. (1985b). *Growing up and growing old in Italian American families*. New Brunswick, NJ: Rutgers University Press.

Johnson, C. L. (1988a). Active and latent functions of grandparenting during the divorce process. *The Gerontologist, 28*, 185–191.

Johnson, C. L. (1988b). *Ex-familia: Grandparents, parents and children adjust to divorce*. New Brunswick, NJ: Rutgers University Press.

Johnson, C. L. (1988c). Postdivorce reorganization of relationships between divorcing children and their parents. *Journal of Marriage and the Family, 50*, 221–231.

Johnson, C. L. (1989). In-law relationships in the American kinship system: Impact of divorce and remarriage. *American Ethnologist, 14*(4), 89–99.

Johnson, C. L. (1995). Cultural diversity in the late-life family. In R. Blieszner & V. H. Bedford (Eds.), *Handbook of aging and the family* (pp. 307–331). Westport, CT: Greenwood Press.

Johnson, C. L., & Barer, B. M. (1987). Marital instability and changing kinship networks of grandparents. *The Gerontologist, 27*(3), 330–335.

Johnson, C. L., & Barer, B. M. (1990). Families and social networks among inner-city Blacks. *The Gerontologist, 30*(6), 726–733.

Johnson, E. S. (1981). Older mothers' perceptions of their child's divorce. *The Gerontologist, 21*, 395–401.

Kahana B., & Kahana, E. (1970). Grandparenthood from the perspective of the developing grandchild. *Developmental Psychology, 3*, 98–105.

Kellam, S. G., Ensminger, M. E., & Turner, R. J. (1977). Family structure and the mental health of children. Concurrent and community-wide studies. *Archives of General Psychiatry, 34*, 1012–1022.

Kennedy, G. E. (1992). Quality in grandparent/grandchild relationships. *International Journal of Aging and Human Development, 35*, 83–98.

Kivett, V. R. (1991). The grandparent-grandchild connection. *Marriage and Family Review, 16*, 267–290.

Kornhaber, A., & Woodward, K. L. (1981). *Grandparents/grandchildren: The vital connection*. Garden City, NY: Doubleday.

Larsen, D. (1991). Grandparent: Redefining the role-unplanned parenthood. *Modern Maturity, 33*(6), 32–36.

Laslett, B. (1978). Family membership, past and present. *Social Problems, 25,* 476–490.

Longfellow, C. (1979). Divorce in context: Its impact on children. In G. Levinger & O. Moles (Eds.), *Divorce and separation* (pp. 287–306). New York: Basic Books.

Longino, C. F., & Earle, T. R. (1996). Who are the grandparents at century's end? *Generations, XX*(1), 13–16.

Lopata, H. Z. (1973). *Widowhood in an American city.* Cambridge, MA: Schenckman.

Markides, K. S., & Mindel, C. H. (1987). *Aging and ethnicity.* Newbury Park, CA: Sage.

Martin, E. P., & Martin, J. M. (1978). *Black extended families.* Chicago: University of Chicago Press.

Matthews, S. H., & Sprey, J. (1984). The impact of divorce on grandparenthood: An exploratory study. *The Gerontologist, 24,* 41–47.

Minkler, M., & Roe, K. M. (1993). *Grandmothers as caregivers: Raising children of the crack cocaine epidemic.* Beverly Hills, CA: Sage.

Minkler, M., & Roe, K. M. (1996). Grandparents as surrogate parents. *Generations, XX*(1), 34–38.

Myers, G. C. (1996). Aging and the social sciences: Research directions and unresolved issues. In R. H. Binstock & L. K. George (Eds.), *Handbook of aging and the social sciences* (4th ed., pp. 1–12). San Diego, CA: Academic Press.

Neugarten, B., & Weinstein, M. (1964). The changing American grandparent. *Journal of Marriage and the Family, 26,* 199–204.

Parsons, T. (1965). The normal American family. In S. Farber (Ed.), *Man and civilization* (pp. 31–50). New York: McGraw-Hill.

Poponoe, D. (1993). The American family decline, 1960–1990: A review and reappraisal. *Journal of Marriage and the Family, 55,* 527–555.

Presser, H. B. (1989). Some economic complexities of child care provided by grandmothers. *Journal of Marriage and the Family, 51,* 581–591.

Preston, S. H. (1984). Children and elders: Divergent paths for America's dependents. *Demography, 21,* 435–457.

Robertson, J. (1977). Grandmotherhood: A study of role conceptions. *Journal of Marriage and the Family, 39,* 165–174.

Robertson, J. F. (1995). Grandparenting in an era of rapid change. In R. Blieszner & V. H. Bedford (Eds.), *Handbook of aging and the family* (pp. 243–260). Westport, CT: Greenwood Press.

Robertson, J., & Johnson, C. L. (1997). Should grandparents assume full parental responsibility? In A. E. Scharlach & L. Kaye (Eds.), *Controversial issues in aging* (pp. 173–184). New York: Allyn & Bacon.

Rossi, A. S., & Rossi, P. H.. (1990). *Of human bonding: Parent-child relations across the life course.* New York: Aldine.

Ruggles, S. (1994). The origins of African-American family structure. *American Sociological Review, 59,* 136–151.

Saluter, A. F. (1992). Marital status and living arrangements: March 1991. *Current population reports, population characteristics.* (Series P–20, No. 461). Washington, DC: U.S. Goverment Printing Office.

Shore, R. J., & Hayslip, B. (1994). Custodial grandparenting: Implications for children's development. In A. E. Gottfried & A. W. Gottfried (Eds.), *Redefining families: Implications for children's development.* New York: Plenum Press.

Simon-Rusinowitz, L., Krach, C. A., Marks, L. N., Piktialis, D., & Wilson, L. B. (1996). Grandparents in the workplace: The effects of economic and labor trends, *Generations, XX*(1), 41–44.

Solomon, J .C., & Marx, J. (1995). "To grandmother's house we go": Health and school adjustment of children raised solely by grandparents. *The Gerontologist, 35,* 386–394.

Spitze, G., Logan, J. R., Deane, G., & Zerger, S. (1994). Adult children's divorce and intergenerational relationships. *Journal of Marriage and the Family, 56,* 279–293.

Sprey, J., & Matthews, S. (1982). Contemporary grandparenthood: A systematic transition. *Annals of the American Academy of Political and Social Science, 464,* 91–103.

Stacy, J. (1993). Good riddance to "The Family": A response to David Poponoe. *Journal of Marriage and the Family, 55,* 545–547.

Staples, R., & Johnson, L. B. (1993). *Black families at the crossroads: Challenges and prospects.* San Francisco, CA: Jossey-Bass.

Thomas, J. L. (1986). Age and sex differences in perceptions of grandparenting. *Journal of Gerontology, 41,* 417–423.

Thompson, L., & Walker, A. (1987). Mothers as mediators of intimacy between grandmothers and their young adult granddaughters. *Family Relations, 36,* 72–77.

Treas, J. (1995). Older Americans in the 1990s and beyond. *Population Bulletin, 50*(2), 2–46.

Troll, L. (1980). Grandparenting. In L. W. Poon (Ed.), *Aging in the 1980s* (pp. 475–484). Washington, DC: American Psychological Association.

Troll, L. (1983). Grandparents: The family watchdogs. In T. Brubaker (Ed.), *Family relationships in later life* (pp. 63–75). Beverly Hills, CA: Sage.

Troll, L. (1994). Family-embedded vs. family-deprived oldest-old: A study of contrasts. *International Journal of Aging and Human Development, 38*(1), 51–64.

Umberson, D. (1992). Relationships between adult children and their parents: Psychological consequences for both generations. *Journal of Marriage and the Family, 54,* 664–674.

Wallerstein, J., & Kelly, J. (1979). Children of divorce: A review. *Social Work, 24,* 468–475.

Weeks, J. R., & Cuellar, J. (1981). The role of family members with helping networks of older people. *The Gerontologist, 21*, 388–394.

Weitzman, L. (1985). *The divorce revolution: The unexpected social and economic consequences for women and children in America*. New York: Free
Press.

White House Conference on Aging. (1995). *Official 1995 White House Conference on Aging: Adopted resolutions*. Washington, DC: White House
Conference on Aging.

White-Means, S. I., & Thornton, M. C. (1990). Labor market choices and home
health care provisions among employed ethnic caregivers. *The Gerontologist,
30*(6), 769–775.

Wilhite, M. (1987). Children, parents and grandparents: Balancing the rights of
association and control. *American Journal of Family Law, 1*, 473–489.

Wilson, M. (1986). The Black extended family: An analytical consideration.
Developmental Psychology, 22, 246–258.

Wood, V., & Robertson, J. (1976). The significance of grandparenthood. In J. F.
Gubrium (Ed.), *Time, roles, and the self in old age* (pp. 278–304). New York:
Human Science Press.

CHAPTER 7

Cultural Aspects of Grandparents Raising Grandchildren: Intergenerational Issues in African-American and Anglo-American Families

Janet C. Mentes

In recent decades, a confluence of social forces has changed the nature of contemporary grandparenthood from a role of indulgent extended kin to a role of surrogate parent for increasing numbers of grandchildren. Census records indicate that in 1994, 3.7 million children coresided with grandparents who were at least partially responsible for their care (Saluter, 1996). These census data of the entire population considerably underestimate the prevalence of grandparental caregiving, especially in minority families (Szinovacz, 1998). Prominent social trends responsible for these changes include the drug and alcohol epidemic in young- to middle-aged adults, the AIDS epidemic, and out-of-wedlock pregnancies among adolescents of both African-Americans and Anglo-Americans. The responses of grandparents to these often devastating social changes support Troll's (1983) concept of grandparent as "family watchdogs" because more grandparents are being called into action to preserve the family during times of crisis. Whereas prior to this time, grandparents had the luxury of serving as figureheads, they now are recruited to help their families at an earlier age because of adolescent pregnancy (Burton & Bengston, 1985; Hagestad & Burton, 1986) and for longer periods of time because of parental drug and alcohol addiction (Burton, 1992; Jendrek, 1993, 1994a; Minkler, Roe, & Price, 1992; Roe, Minkler, Saunders, & Thomson, 1996), parental mental illness (Kelley & Damato, 1995; O'Reilly & Morrison, 1993), and death of a parent who had AIDS (Burnette, 1997). Although these social trends have been viewed as affecting more African-American families, recent literature has indicated that Anglo-American families are affected as well, especially concerning drug and alcohol addiction (Jendrek, 1993, 1994a, 1994b; Kelley, 1993; Kelley & Damato, 1995).

The trend of grandparents caring for grandchildren is of particular interest to nurses, social workers, and other practitioners caring for older persons. A recent demographic profile of grandparents from the 1992–93 National Survey of Families and Households reports that 78% of American grandparents were 55 years of age or older, with 42% of these grandparents age 65 or older (Uhlenberg & Hammill, 1998). Although transition to grandparenthood often occurs during middle age, grandparents who assume full child-rearing responsibilities for their grandchildren, as in the case where parents have died of AIDs, will enter their old age as surrogate parents of adolescent grandchildren. The health consequences of this grandparental parenting role should be a primary concern of all gerontological practitioners as we enter the 21st century.

Although both African- and Anglo-American families are affected by the social forces discussed previously, the family's response to the crisis is tempered by ethnic factors that prescribe family structural characteristics, such as size, intergenerational contact and interaction, and role expectations. A comparison of intergenerational issues between African- and Anglo-American families with reference to how the grandparental caregiving role is enacted will be explored in this chapter. Practice and policy implications for gerontological nurses also will be discussed.

AFRICAN-AMERICAN AND ANGLO-AMERICAN INTERGENERATIONAL ISSUES

Family Structure and Kinship Patterns

Family structure or how the generations in a family align with each other can affect the intergenerational connectedness that a family exhibits, as well as prescribed roles that family members can play. This in turn have an effect on how a grandparent will ultimately enact his or her role within the family. Recently, trends in family structure have been described as varying in width, length, and composition, producing distinctive opportunities for intergenerational contact. These forms are (1) the verticalized or bean pole family (Bengston, Rosenthal, & Burton, 1990), which is a pattern of generational extension with fewer children at any one generation, but four or five generations in existence at the same time; (2) age-condensed (George & Gold, 1991; Ladner & Gourdine, 1984), which is a vertically compact pattern of family structure resulting from consistent patterns of teenage childbearing; (3) truncated (George & Gold); or (4) substitutive (Johnson & Catalano, 1981), which is a structure that evolves when the kin network of the older adult is notably small because of delayed childbearing or childlessness; and (5) reconstituted (George & Gold), which is a pattern of re-formed families that occurs as the result of divorce. Each type of family structure has an effect on the role(s) that its members may play; for example, in the beanpole structure of families, older family members will be in a role for extended periods of time and will be enacting multiple roles at the same time (parent, grandparent, great-grandparent). Further, they will have fewer kin, which often means less support in times of need (Burton & Dilworth-Anderson, 1991). Within the age-condensed pattern where older members are forced to assume roles, like grandparenthood at an earlier age (Burton & Bengston, 1985), the grandparents, often grandmothers, were caught in the middle of the generations giving care to both younger and older generations in their families. At times, they refused to assume the role of grandparent. Within the substitutive structure, older members often substituted remote or fictive kin for support within their network. Finally, within the reconstituted family, opportunities abound for either an extended kin network with grandchildren and in-laws from multiple marriages or a sparse network because of lack of contact with in-laws and grandchildren. This network pattern tends to be regulated by the grandparent's contact with the custodial parent, as well as personal characteristics of the grandparent (Johnson & Barer, 1987).

In examining racial differences, it has been postulated that Anglo-American families have a patrilineal conjugal family focus, with parents assuming a decreasing role in the family life of their adult children, leaving them, as grandparents, in an old conjugal family of two (Parsons, 1943). Anglo-American families tend not to tap collateral kin, like aunts, uncles, and cousins, but tend to turn to parents and grandparents for help or support (Hays & Mindel, 1973). Recent literature has indicated that adult children and their children are moving back in with their parents, often for economic or social reasons (Bengston & Silverstein, 1993). This action reconstructs a multigenerational family structure, often with the grandmother as a pivotal member. Further, although it has been postulated that adult children move away from their families and have limited contact with parents and grandparents, in fact 74% of elderly persons who have an adult child have a child living within a 25-mile radius of them (1987–1988 National Survey of Families and Households, cited in Uhlenberg, 1993). In addition, elderly Anglo-Americans tend to see their children and grandchildren more frequently than African Americans see their families (Mitchell & Register, 1984). In the same study, Uhlenberg further disputes much of the speculation about increased geographic mobility in the current younger generation by presenting statistics that do not show a trend that would produce greater dispersion of kin over time.

By contrast, African-American families historically have been under fire because of their matrifocal pattern (Dodson, 1988; Foster, 1983). Several reasons have been given for this pattern, ranging from the fact that it is an African cultural artifact (Foster) to a contemporary coping mechanism in a society that does not have acceptable marital partners for African-American women (Staples, 1985). Some researchers have postulated that the most important role for an African-American woman is motherhood (Staples) and that the marital relationship is secondary, partially because of the accessibility and supportiveness of the woman's kinship network, which can substitute for a husband's support (Foster). However, all writers indicate that African-American culture does not spurn the two-parent family and marital relationship, but rather the pattern has evolved in direct response to the pressures of racism (Foster; Staples). One might also argue that there is a qualitative difference between a matrifocal family and a single-parent, mother- or grandmother-headed family, the latter being an ethnically expressed value and the former an effect of general social trends outside of the family.

In addition to a prevalent matrifocus in African-American families, Burton and Dilworth-Anderson (1991) looked at the family structures discussed previously. They indicated that African-American families were most likely to exhibit the verticalized, age-condensed, and substitutive patterns of family structure. They emphasized two resultant trends. First, older African Americans are more likely to be a part of four and five generation families and thus simultaneously assume multiple vertical roles (see also Burton, 1996). Second, grandparenthood, which historically has been an important role in extended families, may become increasingly significant as the number of single-parent households increases.

In further exploration of African-American kinship systems, much has been speculated and some information verified through research, that the African-American kinship system is more dense, diverse, and supportive than Anglo-American kinship systems, which tend to be more linear (Burton, 1996; Foster, 1983; Hays & Mindel, 1973; Johnson & Barer, 1990; Markides & Mindel, 1987; Mutran, 1985). Elderly members tend to receive more support from their network, specifically peripheral kin or fictive kin (Johnson & Barer, 1990), as well as offer support to their network by taking in their children and grandchildren (Mitchell & Register, 1984). Socioeconomic effects on kin support also have been explored with mixed results, with one study suggesting that socioeconomic status is more influential than race in explaining whether elderly people give help to their children and grandchildren (Mitchell & Register). This prompts one to look more at individual intra racial differences rather than adhering to the stereotype of African-American family structure when considering the needs of African-American older adults.

Thus through this brief discussion of family structure and kinship patterns, the impact on elderly members, specifically grandparents, can be summarized as follows. Anglo-American elderly persons have a less dense kin network and tend to interact in a more linear fashion with their network, specifically their children and grandchildren (Mitchell & Register, 1984). African-American elderly persons, on the other hand, have denser networks that include fictive kin to whom they can turn when they need support. As always, there are problems in generalization to ethnic and racial groups; thus writers warn about the stereotyping that can occur when looking at all African-American families as being kin rich and supportive (Dodson, 1988; Mitchell & Register). Further, socioeconomic factors may play an important part in kin relationships of both African-American and Anglo-American families.

Timing: On-Time, Off-Time

In the United States, most individuals become grandparents in midlife, with a mean age of 46; however, for African-American women, there is greater variability in the timing of the grandparental role, with as many as one third becoming grandparents in an "off-time" fashion at < 40 years or > 60 years of age (Szinovacz, 1998). This factor highlights the concept of timing of role accession, another factor in the intergenerational issues of families. As Troll (1985) has stated, grandparenthood is a contingent process, one that is dependent on the actions of others. As such, the actual grandparents have little input into the assumption of the role; yet there is an expectation of normative time during adult development, that is, a time-line when a majority of older adults assume the role of grandparent. When the assumption of the grandparental role is too early or too late, the older adult feels out of synchrony with age peers. This event has been referred to as a time-disordered relationship (Seltzer, 1976). Seltzer indicates that the more control an older person feels he or she has over the time-disor-dered event, the less stress will be associated with transition to the role. Since assumption of the grandparental role is largely out of the control of older persons, the disordered timing of the role can cause stress. Several explanations (Hagestad & Burton, 1986) have been offered for why the off-time role transition, especially early transition, to grandparenthood is stressful. First, the grandparent has no time to prepare for the role by reori-enting his or her expectations and other role investments, particularly parental and grandparental role overlap (Szinovacz). Second, when a life transition occurs at the normal, expected time, the experience can be shared with peers, whereas off-time persons may feel deviant and lack social support in the role (Hagestad & Burton). Further, Burton and Bengston (1985) studied African-American grandmothers living in Los Angeles. They found that among the young grandmothers (median age 32), individual previous notions about the role influenced their enactment of the role. Therefore, many of these younger grandmothers, who were often mothers of young children, felt that they were too young to be a grandmother and rejected the role. This rejection of the role had many intergenerational implications for the family, since the young grand-mother's duties were often pushed up a generation and assumed by the great-grandmother.

In a related vein, grandparents may feel off-time when family circum-stances force them to take care of young grandchildren (Burton, 1992; Jendrek, 1993, 1994a; Minkler et al., 1992). There is a sense of regression to an earlier parental role that is out of synchrony with their present life. Many grandparents, particularly in Anglo-American families, tend to reconfigure their relationships with age peers because of the time com-mitment in caring for a grandchild and because they have little in common with friends any longer (Jendrek, 1993, 1994a).

Thus the timing of the grandparenthood has an effect on preparation and enactment of the role, as well as whether the person assuming the role will have the support of age peers. Since the timing of grandparenthood for any given person is dependent on others, the issue of being off-time can be stressful. Becoming a grandparent can be a burden or a source of joy.

AFRICAN-AMERICAN AND ANGLO-AMERICAN GRANDPARENTS AS CAREGIVERS

Grandparents often have supplemented the parental role in both African- and Anglo-American families; however, since the late 1980s, grandparents have been assuming a surrogate parent role with increasing frequency (Szinovacz, 1998). There are a variety of reasons that predispose a grand- parent to take on one of these two subroles (Werner, 1991). The supple- mental role often is enacted to help the parent(s) maintain employment or to help a young adolescent mother cope with a new parental role. The sur- rogate role is most frequently assumed in both African-American and Anglo-American families as a consequence of drug or alcohol abuse or death of the parent of the grandchild (Burnette, 1997; Burton, 1992; Dowdell, 1995; Fuller-Thomson, Minkler, & Driver, 1997; Jendrek, 1993, 1994a; Kelley, 1993; Minkler et al., 1992). A discussion of both subroles will be presented.

Supplemental Role

As mentioned previously, much has been written and assumed about the strong African-American grandmother role in African-American families. Although, historically, African-American grandmothers took on a parental supplemental role to help their children better themselves occupationally as well as to help with young adolescent mothers, one study has indicated that this role may be changing. Burton and Bengston (1985) report on the study of 41 African-American grandmothers, their daughters (new moth- ers), and their mothers (great-grandmothers) who were living in Los Angeles and considered themselves upwardly mobile. The original intent of this study was "to observe the nature of the relationships between both mothers and daughters, and grandmothers and granddaughters when a non-normative (teen and unwed) pregnancy occurred in the family"(p. 62). In the initial stages of the study, a significant unexpected trend occurred: the grandmothers reacted negatively to their new role, not because their daughters were pregnant out of wedlock, but because they themselves were not ready to assume the role of grandmother, which they perceived as a symbol of being old. Several grandmothers completely rejected the role of grandmother. Thus Burton and Bengston examined the issue of timing in accession to the role of grandmother and found that a majority of "off-time" younger grandmothers (median age 32) rejected the role of grandmotherhood, often leaving their mother to take over the role, whereas "on-time" grandmothers (median age 46) felt good about assuming the role and provided supplemental care for their grandchild.

In a later study, Burton (1996) uses two cohorts, an urban and a rural sample of African-American families to compare family role transitions and intergenerational caregiving among aging African-American women. This qualitative study compared caregiving patterns among women in families who experienced normative on-time transitions to parenthood, and thus grandparenthood, with families that experienced early-normative transitions (transitions that were early in terms of the majority culture, but expected transitions for the individual family) and early nonnormative transition. She found that an equitable distribution of caregiving duties for the women across generations existed in the urban families who had normative and early-normative transitions. In families where nonnormative transitions occurred, caregiving duties centered on the young great-grandparent generation, burdening this generation with duties for both younger and older generations. In rural families, a distinct preference for early transition to grandparenthood was exhibited, because it was expected that the grandmother would parent the grandchild, and, therefore, the grandmother had to be sufficiently young to fulfill this task. This pattern of nonadjacent caregiving was further enacted by the new mother, who was expected to take care of her great-grandmother (Burton, 1996).

One important point to consider in looking at this concept of "off-time" is that it has social implications and personal implications. The social implications are related to normative time and when one can be expected to assume the role of grandmother in our society. The personal implications deal with one's own sense of timing regardless of societal expectations and family responsibilities. Thus some of Burton's early grandmothers did embrace the role of grandmother, despite the fact that they had young children themselves. Burton makes one important conclusion: that the role of African-American grandmothers has been largely stereotypic and that timing of entry to the role and competing demands within the multigenerational structure of African-American families affect on the way the grandmother role is enacted. For some African-American families, the role of grandmother is becoming a tenuous role.

Other notable studies have looked at the manner in which poor, urban African-American grandmothers facilitate their adolescent daughters' transition to motherhood (Apfel & Seitz, 1991; Flaherty, 1988; Flaherty, Facteau, & Garver, 1987). Interestingly, none of these studies report the strong rejection of the role of grandmother that Burton's grandmothers did. Perhaps this was due to less representation of younger mothers. Flaherty et al. indicate that the range of ages was 29–59, with a mean age of 42 years, and Apfel & Seitz indicate that their mean age was 39, with a range of 28–55 years. However, the rejection of the grandmother role might be expressed in the types of facilitative roles grandmothers chose to enact.

Methodology for these studies included postpartum field interviews with grandmother and the new mother. Flaherty et al. (1987, p. 67) delineated seven caring functions of African-American grandmothers:

- managing—arranging schedules, activities, and resources
- caretaking—primarily infant care
- coaching—shares beliefs or provides role modeling on how to parent
- assessing—evaluates daughter's attitudes and competency to parent
- nurturing—demonstrates love and emotional support
- assigning—attitudes and behavior reflect ownership of baby
- patrolling—supervises daughter's lifestyle and personal goals

The managing function was the most often assumed function of the grandmothers in the Flaherty et al. study (1987). Further, they found that grandmothers encouraged their daughters to care for their infants and supported their daughters' efforts to continue with school.

Apfel and Seitz (1991) developed four conceptual models of familial adaptation to adolescent parenthood. Through field interviews, they studied 119 African-American inner-city adolescent first-time mothers and their mothers or surrogate mothers. The four conceptual models discerned were: (1) parental replacement model, where the grandmother takes over parenting of the grandchild; (2) parental supplement model, where the grandmother and other kin share responsibility for care of the grandchild; (3) supported primary parent model, where the mother has the responsibility for care of the child with some support from grandmother; and (4) the parental apprenticeship model, where the grandmother acts as a mentor to her daughter, whom she views as an apprentice. Having delineated these models, the authors state that they have usefulness in medical, school, and social service settings as a reference for intervening to support adaptive coping and perhaps to educate grandmothers about alternate models for supporting their daughter's mothering efforts.

As a part of a study to look at all grandparents who care for their grandchildren, Jendrek (1993, 1994a) examined the day care that Anglo-American grandparents in Ohio provided for their grandchildren. Grandparents provided this care to their very young grandchildren (newborn–3years of age) so that their children could work, and, as such, the role is part-time on a daily basis and usually ends when the child goes to school. Therefore, the assumption of the role has less impact on the grandparents' lifestyle. Further, day care provided by grandparents is a hidden service in that most (81%) grandparents provide the care in their own homes and most (71%) are not paid for the care they give.

Surrogate Role

There has been a dramatic increase in the number of grandchildren living with their grandparents in the last 10 years. In 1994, 3.7 million children in the United States lived with grandparents (Saluter, 1996). This represents a 44% increase since 1980. African-American children (12.1%) are much more likely than Anglo-American children (3.7%) to live with grandparents, but the rate of Anglo-American children represents a 54% increase (Saluter, 1992, 1996).

Much of the increase in coresidence between grandparents and grandchildren has been attributed to the crack cocaine epidemic for African-American families (Burton, 1992; Minkler et al., 1992; Roe et al., 1996; Seamon, 1992), to drug and alcohol problems in Anglo-American families (Jendrek, 1993, 1994a; Kelley, 1993), and to the AIDS/HIV epidemic for both (Burnette, 1997; Joslin & Brouard, 1995; Kelley & Damato, 1995). As a result of this increase, caretaker grandparents are being studied much like other caregivers, with a concern about the burden of caregiving.

As with other caregiving roles, the decision to assume the role is fraught with stress, guilt, and health consequences. Thus much of the current literature is exploratory and descriptive in nature and looks at the stressors and health effects of parenting grandchildren. Several articles make suggestions for service provision and policy changes to help grandparents manage their surrogate parental role. The studies to be discussed focus mostly on grandmothers who are in their mid-50s who have taken on the care of their grandchildren because of parental drug abuse. Burton (1992), Joslin and Brouard (1995); Minkler, Fuller-Thomson, Miller, and Driver

(1997); Minkler et al. (1992), Roe et al. (1996), and Seamon (1992) studied African-American grandmothers in urban areas, whereas Jendrek (1994a), Kelley (1993), and Morrow-Kondos, Weber, Cooper, and Hesser (1997) looked at Anglo-American grandmothers and grandfathers in Ohio, the Northeast, and the Southwest. Dowdell (1995) had a relatively evenly distributed sample (58% African-American grandmothers, 38% Anglo-American grandmothers), but she did not look at racial differences.

Stressors that caregiving grandparents reported tended to fit into three levels that Burton (1992) determined in her two studies of urban African-American grandmothers. These levels included contextual, familial, and individual stressors. She indicated that for her sample, *contextual stressors* were those related to a high-crime, drug-traffic-field neighborhood; the *familial stressors* were those related to the care of multiple kin and drains on the family income; and finally, *individual stressors* were those that related to balancing multiple roles while not having time for self. Using Burton's conceptualizations, other studies' stressors can be summarized in Table 7.1.

In addition to stressors, the issue of how caregiving affected grandmothers' health was an area of study. Although most grandmothers caring for grandchildren reported that they were in fair-to-good physical health, they also reported that they had postponed their own medical care in response to caregiving needs (Roe et al., 1996). Most grandparental caregivers reported emotional difficulties because of the caregiving role; these ranged from emotional strain (Minkler et al., 1992) to near clinical depression in 44% of grandparents, as measured by the Symptom Checklist-90 in Kelley's study (1993). In a recent national study, Minkler et al. (1997) found that grandparents who provide primary care for a grandchild were twice as likely to have increased depressive symptoms, as measured on the Center for Epidemiological Studies Depression Scale (CES-D). Further, undertaking the care of a grandchild was associated with increased risk for depression among those who recently assumed the role: women, younger grandparents, and those in poor physical health (Minkler et al., 1997). Burton (1992) also noted pervasive effects on the health of her grandparents in that 86% reported that they felt depressed or anxious most of the time, 61% increased their levels of smoking, 38% increased levels of alcohol intake, and 38% reported an increase in physical problems related to diabetes and hypertension. Thus these grandmothers were stressed by their surrogate role responsibilities; however, the majority of grandmothers also acknowledged the importance of the role. Some even indicated that their grandchildren kept them young, and they revised health habits to improve

TABLE 7.1 Stressors Associated With Raising Grandchildren According to Burton's Framework

Contextual
- Paid work mimics caregiving role at home (Minkler et al., 1992)
- Fear of continued maltreatment of grandchildren if parents gain custody (Kelley, 1993)
- Concern for personal safety in neighborhood (Seamon, 1992)

Familial
- Combined caregiving to grandchildren and to elderly relatives, feeling helpless to help child who has drug problem (Minkler et al., 1992; Roe et al., 1996)
- Fear that child will inherit parent's substance abuse problem (Kelley, 1993)
- Caregiver stress, lack of support and resources (Seamon, 1992)
- Financial concerns, lack of family support (Dowdell, 1995)
- Disappoinment and guilt in dealing with their adult child (Morrow-Kondos et al., 1997)

Individual
- Hoped for a more tenuous grandparental role (Minkler et al., 1992)
- Fear that will not live long enough to raise the grandchild (Kelley, 1993)
- Poor physical health and unmarried (Dowdell, 1995)
- Fatigue (Morrow-Kondos et al., 1997)

their health so that they would better ensure that they could see their grandchild to adulthood (Minkler et al.,1992; Morrow-Kondos et al., 1997).

Finally, Jendrek (1993) looked at the effect of different levels (custodial, living with, day care) of grandparental caregiving on lifestyle; she did not measure physical or emotional health as such. She did find that custodial grandparents, those who had legal custody of their grandchildren, suffered more drastic lifestyle changes that involved less contact with friends, less time for spouse, less personal time, more need to alter plans, and increased feelings of physical and emotional tiredness.

Grandparents at all levels also acknowledged that they had an increased sense of purpose in their lives since caring for their grandchildren. Thus, although caring for a grandchild was stressful for both African-American and Anglo-American grandparents, there was a positive side that partially offset the negative consequences of caregiving.

IMPLICATIONS FOR GERONTOLOGICAL NURSES

Practice Issues

Although nurses of several specialty areas should be aware of the issues surrounding grandparents as caregivers to their grandchildren, this section will focus on gerontological nurses. Burnette (1997) aptly points out that any professional working with these grandparents and their families must have knowledge not only of aging, but of child welfare, substance abuse, HIV/AIDS infection, and legal issues as well. It is important for gerontological nurses to take a comprehensive view when working with caregiving grandparents, since much of the distress that they may be experiencing is related to the welfare of their grandchildren.

In fact, gerontological nurse practitioners (GNPs) who work in primary care settings should be aware of the health consequences of grandparental parenting and be prepared to meet special needs through education and counseling. This may be a particularly difficult population to treat, especially if they postpone or cancel regular health care visits. The GNP may have to make home visits to make a complete assessment and offer appropriate treatment. In addition, the GNP could well be the first health professional to detect depressive symptoms in these caregivers and should be aware that grandparents who have recently assumed the caregiving role are at increased risk for depression (Minkler et al., 1997; Strawbridge, Wallhagen, Shema, & Kaplan, 1997). Hence, inquiring about caregiving activities should be part of every health visit.

Given the high level of stress cited in many of the studies, counseling and support groups for grandparents raising grandchildren are essential. In the past 5 years, support organizations for grandparents have formed in many states, with the AARP Grandparent Information Center serving as a prototype organization (Kelley & Damato, 1995). Interested nurses could initiate support groups for grandparents as a part of their job responsibilities in hospital and community settings. Focus of the group should include discussing caregiving stressors as well as providing information on current financial and legal issues affecting grandparent caregivers (Flint & Perez-Porter, 1997).

A preventive activity that nurses can provide is grandparent education, which could empower grandparent caregivers by helping them to anticipate and plan for potential problems that occur as a result of being a caregiver to grandchildren. This concept is supported by the fact that more than 40% of first-time grandparents, particularly African-American grand-parents, indicate that they could benefit from educational programs to help them adapt to the role (Watson & Koblinsky, 1997). Strom, Collinsworth, Strom, and Griswold (1993) describe an educational program titled "Becoming a Better Grandparent," which was developed for African Americans and focused on developmental needs of their grandchildren, such as how to devote more conversations to topics that interest their grandchildren, promote problem solving as a way to help adolescent grandchildren avoid obstacles to a successful future, and support educational opportunities of grandchildren.

Grandparent education for the supplemental role of grandmothers who are helping their teenage daughters learn how to mother, as suggested by Apfel & Seitz (1991), could be implemented by teams of pediatric and gerontological nurses. The gerontological nurse can serve as a coach for the grandmother who is learning appropriate skills to model the role and support her daughter in her new role as mother, rather than assume parental duties. Careful ethnic assessment must be accomplished prior to initiating an educational program of this sort, because for some ethnic groups, such as the rural African-American families described by Burton (1996), this program may undermine their normative role functions.

Policy Issues

Gerontological nurses, as patient advocates, need to support changes in public policy that would benefit custodial grandparents. Financial and legal issues tend to be significant stressors for grandparents caring for their grandchildren, with 25% of them living below the poverty line (Fuller-Thomson et al., 1997). This fact, in combination with a social welfare system that often sabotoges kin care of these children by forcing grandparents to formally adopt or enter the foster care system to receive financial aid for their care, is extremely stressful for low-income grandparents (Burnette, 1997; Flint & Perez-Porter, 1997). In addition, grandparents receiving welfare because they have left jobs to care for grandchildren are in jeopardy of losing benefits with the passage of the Personal Responsibility and Work Opportunity Reconciliation Act of 1996 (PRA), which limits benefits to a 60-month limit (Burnette). Individual states can choose to continue to provide benefits for these grandparents or establish other mechanisms to support grandparents raising their grandchilden.

Another policy issue relates to health insurance coverage for grandchildren (Jendrek, 1994b). As previously discussed, many of these grandparent-headed families have limited financial resourses, and so they may forgo their own health needs to meet their grandchildrens' needs. This is especially so in families where the grandchild may have extensive health needs because of prenatal drug exposure. Although grandparents and grandchildren may qualify for Medicaid coverage or Supplemental Security Income, these benefits are subject to the PRA and therefore may be discontinued. Even though grandparent caregivers above 65 years of age would qualify for Medicare for their own health care, less than a quarter of all grandparents meet that age criterion (Burnette, 1997). In addition, private health insurance does not cover grandchildren unless they are formally adopted, which usually does not occur, especially in African-American families (Burnette).

Finally, nurses should advocate for the provision of respite services and support groups for grandparents who are caring for their grandchildren. This may be accomplished by providing these services through Areas on Aging or expanding services supported by the AARP, which has been active in the support of these grandparents.

Research Issues

Grandparenthood offers some interesting areas for nursing research. Nursing has done an exceptional job of exploring caregiving relationships of caregivers of elderly family members, specifically those with Alzheimer's disease. A logical extension of that research focus would be with grandparents caring for healthy grandchildren or special needs grandchildren because of the effects of parental drug or alcohol use. How do these caregiving situations differ? Additional information also is needed about the African-American caregivers and the contemporary African-American family. Have the family kinship relations changed thereby affecting the experience of grandparenting? How do middle-class African-American grandparents fit into this picture? And how can nurses improve the physical and emotional health of caregiving grandparents? These are just a few topics that might be of interest for a program of nursing research.

CONCLUSION

An attempt has been made to explore how African-American and Anglo-American intergenerational issues affect grandparents as caregivers. The issue of race seemed to be most significant when looking at intergenerational family issues, specifically family structure and kinship relations. Although African-American families often have been labeled as pathologic or deviant, much of the literature reviewed pointed more to the fact that African-American families and their elderly grandparental generation were resilient and had adapted well in a hostile environment. The richness of African-American family kin networks as compared to Anglo-American families was evident in a number of studies; however, these same studies pointed to the need to not overgeneralize about African-American families to the extent that they do not receive any formal support. In fact, African-American families and their elderly members benefit from a combination of informal and formal supports.

In consideration of African-American and Anglo-American grandparents as caregivers, the differences in need become less apparent in that Anglo- and African-American grandparents evidenced similar issues in caring for grandchildren. However, although needs are similar between these two groups of caregiving grandparents, recent research has indicated that African-American grandparents are twice as likely to become caregivers for their grandchildren than are Anglo-American grandparents (Fuller-Thomson et al., 1997), necessitating further research into this area and provision of culturally sensitive care.

REFERENCES

Apfel, N., & Seitz, V. (1991). Four models of adolescent mother-grandmother relationships in African-American inner-city families. *Family Relations, 40,* 421–429.

Bengston, V., Rosenthal, C., & Burton, L. (1990). Families and aging: Diversity and heterogeneity. In R. Binstock & L. George (Eds.), *Handbook of aging and the social sciences* (3rd ed., pp. 263–287). San Diego, CA: Academic Press.

Bengston, V., & Silverstein, M. (1993). Families, aging, and social change: Seven agendas for 21st century. *Annual Review of Gerontology and Geriatrics, 13,* 15–38.

Burnette, D. (1997). Grandparents raising grandchildren in the inner city. *Families in Society: Journal of Contemporary Human Services, 78*(5), 489–499.

Burton, L. (1992). African-American grandparents rearing children of drug-addicted parents: Stressors, outcomes, and social service needs. *The Gerontologist, 32,* 744–751.

Burton, L. (1996). Age norms, the timing of family role transitions and intergenerational caregiving among aging African-American women. *The Gerontologist, 36*(2), 199–208.

Burton, L., & Bengston, V. (1985). African-American grandmothers. Issues of timing and continuity of roles. In V. Bengston & J. Robertson (Eds.), *Grandparenthood* (pp. 61–77). Beverly Hills, CA: Sage.

Burton, L., & Dilworth-Anderson, P. (1991). The intergenerational family roles of aged African-American Americans. *Marriage and Family Review, 16*, 311–330.

Dodson, J. (1988). Conceptualizations of African-American families. In H. McAdoo (Ed.), *African-American families* (pp. 77–90). Newbury Park, CA: Sage.

Dowdell, E. (1995). Caregiver burden: Grandmothers raising their high risk grandchildren. *Journal of Psychosocial Nursing, 33*(3), 27–30.

Flaherty, M. (1988). Seven caring functions of African-American grandmothers in adolescent mothering. *Journal of Maternal Child Health Nursing, 17*, 191–207.

Flaherty, M., Facteau, L., & Garver, P. (1987). Grandmother functions in multi-generational families: An exploratory study of African-American adolescent mothers and their infants. *Journal of Maternal Child Nursing, 16*, 61–73.

Foster, H. (1983). African patterns in the Afro-American family. *Journal of African-American Studies, 14*(2), 201–232.

Fuller-Thomson, E., Minkler, M., & Driver, D. (1997). A profile of grandparents raising grandchildren in the United States. *The Gerontologist, 37*(3), 406–411.

George, L., & Gold, D. (1991). Life course perspectives on intergenerational connections. *Marriage and Family Review, 16*, 67–88.

Grant, R., Gordon, S. G., & Cohen, S. T. (1997). An innovative school-based intergenerational model to serve grandparent caregivers. *Journal of Gerontological Social Work, 28*, 1–2, 47–61.

Hagestad, G., & Burton, L. (1986). Grandparenthood, life context, and family development. *American Behavioral Scientist, 29*, 471–484.

Hays, W., & Mindel, C. (1973). Extended kinship relations in African-American and Anglo-American families. *Journal of Marriage and Family, 35*, 51–57.

Jendrek, M. (1993). Grandparents who parent their grandchildren: Effects on lifestyle. *Journal of Marriage and the Family, 55*, 609–621.

Jendrek, M. (1994a). Grandparents who parent their grandchildren: Circumstances and decisions. *The Gerontologist, 34*, 206–216.

Jendrek, M. (1994b). Policy concerns of Anglo-American grandparents who provide regular care to their grandchildren. *Journal of Gerontological Social Work, 32*, 175–200.

Johnson, C., & Barer, B. (1987). Marital instability and the changing kinship networks of grandparents. *The Gerontologist, 27*, 330–335.

Johnson, C., & Barer, B. (1990). Families and networks among older inner-city African-Americans. *The Gerontologist, 30,* 726–733.

Johnson, C., & Catalano, D. (1981). Childless elderly and their family support. *The Gerontologist, 21,* 610–618.

Joslin, D., & Brouard, A. (1995). The prevalence of grandmothers as primary caregivers in a poor pediatric population. *Journal of Community Health, 20*(5), 383–401.

Kelley, S. (1993). Caregiver stress in grandparents raising grandchildren. *Image, 25,* 331–337.

Kelley, S., & Damato, E. (1995). Grandparents as primary caregivers. *Maternal Child Nursing, 20,* 326–332.

Ladner, J., & Gourdine, R. (1984). Intergenerational teenage motherhood: Some preliminary findings. *Sage: A Scholarly Journal on African-American Women, 1*(2), 22–24.

Markides, K., & Mindel, C. (1987). *Aging and ethnicity* (pp. 97–120). Newbury Park, CA: Sage.

Minkler, M., Fuller–Thomson, E., Miller, M., & Driver, D. (1997). Depression in grandparents raising grandchildren. Results of a national longitudinal study. *Archives of Family Medicine, 6,* 445–452.

Minkler, M., Roe, K., & Price, M. (1992). The physical and emotional health of grandmothers raising grandchildren in the crack cocaine epidemic. *The Gerontologist, 32,* 752–761.

Mitchell, J., & Register, J. (1984). An exploration of family interaction with the elderly by race, socioeconomic status and residence. *The Gerontologist, 24,* 48–54.

Morrow-Kondos, D., Weber, J., Cooper, K., & Hesser, J. (1997). Becoming parents again: Grandparents raising grandchildren. *Journal of Gerontological Social Work, 28*(1/2), 35–46.

Mutran, E. (1985). Intergenerational family support among blacks and whites: Response to culture or to socioeconomic differences. *Journal of Gerontology, 40,* 382–389.

O'Reilly, E., & Morrison, M. L. (1993). Grandparent-headed families: New therapeutic challenges. *Child Psychiatry and Human Development, 23*(3), 147–159.

Parsons, T. (1943). The kinship system of the contemporary United States. *American Anthropologist, 45,* 22–38.

Roe, K., Minkler, M., Saunders, F., & Thomson, G. (1996). Health of grandmothers raising children of the crack cocaine epidemic. *Medical Care, 34*(11), 1072–1084.

Saluter, A. (1992, March). Marital status and living arrangements: *Current Population Reports*, (Series P-20, No. 468). U.S. Bureau of the Census. Washington, DC: U.S. Government Printing Office.

Saluter, A. (1996, March). Marital status and living arrangements: *Current Population Reports*, (Series P20–491). U.S. Bureau of the Census, Washington, DC: U.S. Government Printing Office.

Seamon, F. (1992). Intergenerational issues related to the crack cocaine problem. *Family and Community Health, 15*(3), 11–19.

Seltzer, M. (1976). Suggestions for the examination of time-disordered relationships. In J. F. Gubrium (Ed.), *Time, roles and self in old age* (pp. 111–125). New York: Human Science Press.

Staples, R. (1985). Changes in African-American family structure: The conflict between family ideology and structural conditions. *Journal of Marriage and the Family, 47*, 1005–1013.

Strawbridge, W., Wallhagen, M., Shema, S., & Kaplan, G. (1997). New burdens or more of the same? Comparing grandparent, spouse and adult child caregivers. *The Gerontologist, 37*(4), 505–510.

Strom, R., Collinsworth, P., Strom, S., & Griswold, D. (1993). Strengths and needs of African-American grandparents. *International Journal of Aging and Human Development, 36*, 255–268.

Szinovacz, M. (1998). Grandparents today: A demographic profile. *The Gerontologist, 38*(1), 37–52.

Troll, L. (1983). Grandparents: The family watchdogs. In T. Brubaker (Ed.), *Family relationships in later life* (pp. 63–74). Beverly Hills, CA: Sage.

Troll, L. (1985). The contingencies of grandparenting. In V. Bengston & J. Robertson (Eds.), *Grandparenthood* (pp. 135–149). Beverly Hills, CA: Sage.

Uhlenberg, P. (1993). Demographic change and kin relationships in later life. *Annual Review of Gerontology and Geriatrics, 13*, 219–238.

Uhlenberg, P., & Hammill, B. (1998). Frequency of grandparent contact with grandchild sets: Six factors that make a difference. *The Gerontologist, 38*(3), 276–285.

Watson, J., & Koblinsky, S. (1997). Strengths and needs of working-class African-American and Anglo-American grandparents. *International Journal of Aging and Human Development, 44*(2), 149–165.

Werner, E. (1991). Grandparent-grandchild relationships amongst U.S. ethnic groups. In P. Smith (Ed.), *The psychology of grandparenthood* (pp. 68–82). New York: Rutledge.

CHAPTER 8

Legal and Ethical Issues for Older Adults in Transition

Kay Weiler and Perle Slavik Cowen

Modern medical technology has dramatically increased life expectancy resulting in protracted periods of time during which elderly persons are susceptible to physical and cognitive impairments and subsequently have greater dependency needs (Council on Scientific Affairs, 1987). In 1994 there were 33.2 million elderly Americans (age 65 or older) comprising one eighth of the country's population (Bureau of the Census, 1996). Among this group, 18.7 million were ages 65 to 74, 11 million were 75 to 84, and 3.5 million were 85 or older. The "oldest old" (persons age 85 and above) are the most rapidly growing segment with a 274% increase since 1960, while the population of those 65 and above has doubled. It is predicted that by the middle of the next century, the number of persons 65 years old and older will more than double to 80 million, while the "oldest old" population is expected to double in size by 2020, reaching a total of 7 million persons that year (Hobbs & Damon, 1996).

Advances in health care have produced mechanisms for extending the quantity of life; however, frail elderly people may not be experiencing the same general physical health that might have been experienced by the previous old age survivors (Steinmetz, 1990). Health professionals have reported that recent cost-containment measures, implemented by hospitals in response to Medicare Diagnosis Related Groups (DRGs), have resulted in the vulnerable elderly person being discharged "quicker and sicker" and that such practices represent a form of societal and institutional mistreatment

(Baumhover, Beall, & Pieroni, 1990). The current trends in smaller family size and more blended families have resulted in fewer numbers of offspring who must share responsibility for their own elderly parents and relatives from current and previous marriages (Steinmetz, 1990). These family members often are novices in providing complex physical care and are not prepared for the long-term consequences of caring for an elder family member (Boland & Sims, 1996) especially since most have little involvement in decisions to discharge the family member from care in a hospital (Sims, Boland, & O'Neill, 1992).

Both the increasing numbers and longevity of older adults have broad societal implications regarding how we can adequately address their changing needs. Accompanying the increases in age are increasing needs for personal assistance with ADLs and potentially decreasing decision-making abilities. The changes may precipitate a change in standard of living, location of residence (single family dwelling, in-home care, assisted living or long-term care facilities) and a need for increasing intensity of care for those who become technology dependent. The changes also may precipitate changes in their actual decision-making skills or others' perceptions of their decision-making ability.

Many of the changes associated with aging are accompanied by legal and ethical issues that the elderly persons and those who are concerned about them must consider. To examine relevant issues for elderly persons, this chapter will use four ethical principles: autonomy, beneficence, nonmaleficence, and justice. Appropriate legal considerations will be integrated into each of the four ethical concerns.

ETHICAL CONCEPTS AND LEGAL APPLICATIONS

Autonomy

Autonomy is usually described as the right of self-governance or self-determination. Autonomy may, however, be the interaction of various aspects that facilitate self-governance, such as: (1) liberty of action; (2) freedom of choice; or (3) effective deliberation (Mappes & Zembaty, 1986). When autonomy is viewed as liberty of action, it identifies that the individual's actions are the result of a conscious decision to voluntarily act in a specific manner. The individual is not coerced into action by the use of force or the threat of force. Autonomy as freedom of choice indicates that the individual has the right to choose which option(s) he or she prefers for the specific situation. The options may be very limited, e.g., surgery or chemotherapy as treatment for a terminal illness. However, the patient is not being limited because he or she is coerced into a specific decision. The limitations exist because of the restricted number of alternatives available for the specific situation. Effective deliberation is another aspect of autonomy that includes an individual's ability to make rational and unconstrained decisions and then act according to those decisions. This aspect of autonomy is based upon the premise that actions follow deliberation (Mappes & Zembaty, 1986).

To exercise autonomy, an individual must have the decision-making capacity to make decisions, voluntarily act, and choose the option(s) that he or she prefers. Within the legal domain, decision-making ability is generally referred to as mental competency. The determination regarding whether or not an individual has legal competency is generally very simple—all adults are presumed competent. The concept of competency, however, has limited usefulness if an individual retains the status of an adult but has decreased or no decision-making capacity or has lost the ability to care for him or herself due to various cognitively incapacitating experiences (Willis, 1996).

The terminology "decision-making capacity" is frequently used by health care professionals who have concluded that discussions or assessments of decision-making capacity are much more useful measures of decision-making ability than the legal term of competency. Decision-making capacity may be described as the ability "to understand the nature and effects of one's acts" (Aiken & Catalano, 1994). Or capacity may be defined as requiring a set of personal values or goals; the ability to communicate and understand information; and the ability to deliberate and reason regarding the available options (Northrop & Kelly, 1987). Decision-making incapacity in an adult may be determined by one or a combination of several criteria: the presence of a disabling condition; the lack of ability to make and communicate cognitive decision making; the inability to meet his or her essential needs; and the personal endangerment by the lack of decision-making capacity (Smyer, Schaie, & Kapp, 1996). Once the distinction between the legal concept of competency and the functional status of decision-making capacity is accepted, it is clearly possible that an adult may retain the legal presumption of competency; however, the individual may not have the decision-making capacity to make essential decisions regarding safety, security, or health care.

Informed Consent

An adult's primary expression of autonomy within the health care system is the requirement that adults must give "informed" consent before any treatment is initiated (*Schloendorff v. Society of New York Hospital*, 1914). Each state has the authority to determine what criteria must be met in that state to establish that the patient was appropriately informed about the anticipated intervention. Generally, the laws require: (1) the patient must have decision-making capacity; (2) the decision is voluntarily made; (3) there is an informational process; and (4) the risks and benefits of the pro- posed treatment are disclosed and discussed (Brent, 1997). It is important to remember that an individual's right to give an informed consent includes the right to give an informed refusal to care (*Cruzan v. Director, Missouri Department of Health*, 1990). As the person transitions from middle adulthood into the elderly years, health status may change or decline, and health care professionals have a heightened obligation to monitor the individuals' decision-making capacity and their ability to rec- ognize the ramifications of their current health care needs.

An individual's right to consent to or refuse care is not absolute (Aiken & Catalano, 1994). It is balanced against four other competing social inter- ests: the preservation of human life; the prevention of suicide; the protec- tion of the interests of innocent third parties; and the preservation of the integrity of the medical profession (*Brophy v. New England Sinai Hospital*, Inc., 1986).

There are very few exceptions to the health care professional's obliga- tion to provide the patient with the information required for an informed consent. These exceptions include therapeutic privilege, waiver, emer- gency and unanticipated events (Aiken & Catalano, 1994). Therapeutic privilege occurs when the health care provider believes that the patient would be physically or psychologically harmed if the relevant information were disclosed. A waiver to informed consent occurs when the patient has clearly identified a desire not to receive relevant information. An emer- gency exception to informed consent doctrine includes the responsibility to intervene, without consent, if the patient's life is in jeopardy. Finally, the unanticipated events exception generally arises during surgical procedures where an unanticipated condition is encountered and if it is not acted upon, the condition could expose the patient to increased health risks or neces- sitate a second surgery after a more specific informed consent was obtained (Aiken & Catalano, 1994; U.S. Congress, 1987). A potential extension of the right to consent or right to refuse health care (*Cruzan v.*

Director, Missouri Department of Health, 1990) has been identified as the right to request care that will result in the person's death or assisted suicide (*Vacco v. Quill*, 1997).

Advanced Planning for Decisions Regarding Personal or Health Care

In the past, there were no legal mechanisms that protected the adult's right to determine in advance what he or she might want for future health care. The adult relied on immediate family members or the personal local physician to follow what seemed "best" in the given situation. This mechanism was only effective if the family members or physician survived the adult and if the family or physician sincerely had the best interests of the patient in forming the treatment decision. Today, however, there has been a transition within the legal system that has created the need to formulate documents that express an individual's wishes for future health care needs.

The legal system has identified situations that may occur and leave the adult with legal competency but little, if any, decision-making capacity. The law has provisions in which one adult may make a substitute or surrogate decision of another adult in need of care. In essence the surrogate decision maker asserts the impaired adult's autonomy by making substituted decisions on behalf of the impaired adult. The titles and purposes of the substitute decision makers vary depending on who has initiated the appointment of the substitute decision maker and the scope of authority that has been delegated to the substitute decision maker. Specifically, there are some situations in which an adult, who retains competency and capacity, may make a current designation of another person to make financial, health care, or personal care decisions if the declaring adult becomes incapacitated in the future (Hall, 1996). If these delegations of authority are specifically for future health care treatment decisions, they are referred to as advance directives and are generally classified as a living will or a durable power of attorney for health care (Hall, 1996; Teno et al., 1997). If the adult has moved from having decision-making capacity to having lost this capacity, the surrogate decision maker is court appointed and generally referred to as a guardian (Schuster, 1996).

Living Will (LW)

Adults may progress through varied conditions or situations that emphasize the individual's need for advanced health care planning (e.g., death of a parent or sibling, diagnosis of a chronic illness). The LW provides adults the opportunity to describe any life sustaining treatment they wish to accept or reject if they experience a terminal condition or permanent state of unconsciousness and are not able to participate in health care treatment decisions. This document is the individual's own statement of preferences for future health care. Almost all states have LW legislation, and although each state has the authority to draft legislation applicable only to the residents of that state, the legal and ethical principles of personal autonomy are the premises of each law (Krauskopf, Brown, & Tokarz, 1996). Typical criteria for LW statutes include: (1) the individual is an adult; (2) who has lost the capacity to participate in the necessary health care treatment decision; (3) has a terminal illness or a condition that is not considered curable (e.g., persistent vegetative state); and (4) requires life-sustaining treatment (Uniform Rights of the Terminally Ill Act, 1985).

Durable Power of Attorney for Health Care (DPAHC)

The LW discussed above is limited to life-sustaining procedures. However, many important health care treatment decisions are not covered by the narrow parameters of a LW. Therefore, the individual should consider the appointment of a DPAHC, which may be useful in a variety of specific transitions within the aging process (e.g., a need for monitored living arrangements or access to complex technological equipment with qualified health care professionals). A DPAHC is a private legal relationship that is created by a document in which one person (the principal) grants another person (the agent, surrogate, proxy, or attorney-in-fact) the authority to act for him or her in making personal or health care treatment decisions. This delegation of authority continues even if the principal becomes cognitively incapacitated. This relationship has the advantage of authorizing a designated person to receive pertinent diagnostic information, analyze potential treatment options, act as an advocate for the patient, and give consent for or refusal of care. Forty nine states and the District of Columbia have a proxy decision-maker for health care treatment decisions (Krauskopf, Brown, & Tokarz, 1996).

All 50 states have legislation recognizing either LW or DPAHC options (Choice in Dying, 1994). In an attempt to increase public awareness of the legal options available for health care treatment decisions, encourage compliance with stated treatment preferences, and provide significant penalties for those who do not comply, the federal legislature enacted the Patient Self-Determination Act (PSDA).

The Patient Self-Determination Act (1990)

The previously mentioned Act requires every health care institution to maintain specific policies and procedures for every adult who receives health care in that institution. Failure to comply with the Act may result in a facility's loss of Medicare and Medicaid payments. The policies were drafted for the following reasons:

(A) to provide written information to each such individual concerning:
  (i) an individual's rights under State law (whether statutory or as recognized by the courts of the State) to make decisions concerning such medical care, including the right to accept or refuse medical or surgical treatment and the right to formulate advance directives...
  (ii) the written policies of the provider or organization respecting the implementation of such rights.

(B) to document in the individual's medical record whether or not the individual has executed an advance directive.

The creation of the Patient Self-Determination Act was the direct result of the court battle that Nancy Cruzan's parents waged in to have her gastrostomy tube feedings discontinued. Nancy was a 26-year-old woman who had decision-making capacity until she was involved in a serious automobile accident and was thrown, face down, into a puddle of water. After suffering anoxia for a projected period of 15 minutes, Nancy never regained the ability to interact with her environment and was adjudicated to lack decision-making capacity regarding any personal care decisions. Older adults are certainly at risk of automobile accidents, cerebral vascular accidents, or trauma, which may suddenly propel them into a health care status that, temporarily or permanently, deprives the adults of their decision-making capacity.

Advanced Planning for Decisions Regarding Financial Concerns

One of the most frequently expressed concerns by elderly persons is the change in financial status that may occur with retirement, the death of a spouse, or increased financial needs due to special diets or medications. There are multiple options that may be available for planning for future financial needs. Some of the options may be limited to those who have significant financial resources (trust), or those who have a trusted friend or family member (e.g., durable power of attorney or joint tenancy). In the following paragraphs, a the variety of options for assisting elders during this transitional period are presented.

Durable Power of Attorney

The durable power of attorney is one legal mechanism that may be written to provide a very limited or extensive delegation of financial decision-making authority. A durable power of attorney is a private written document in which the elderly person (the principal) has granted another person (the agent or attorney-in-fact) the authority to act for him or her. This legal principle of delegation of authority to another person is the historical precedent that served as the model for the DPAHC described previously (Strauss & Lederman, 1996) However, it is important to note that the durable power of attorney is limited to the delegation of authority for financial transactions (e.g., purchase or sale of property, execution of a contract) and does not extend to personal or health care treatment decisions (Strauss & Lederman, 1996).

The historical common law form of a power of attorney required that the principal have cognitive decision-making ability at the initiation of the relationship and retain that decision-making capacity for the duration of the relationship. If the principal lost decision-making capacity, the delegation of authority from the principal to the agent became void. This requirement for continued capacity indicated that this delegation of authority was not useful for individuals who wanted to plan for future decision-making incapacity or who anticipated progressively declining decision-making capacity, e.g. Alzheimer's disease (Strauss & Lederman, 1996).

The *durable* power of attorney was created to meet the needs of individuals who wanted to have the delegation of authority continue even if the principal experienced changes in decision-making capacity. The agent in a *durable* power of attorney relationship continues to have the legal authority to act for the principal even if the principal has no decision-making capacity.

The most significant disadvantages of the durable power of attorney relationship are the limited safeguards available to the principal or elderly person. If the agent is not acting in the principal's best interests or is misappropriating the principal's funds, the principal may revoke the agreement. However, the agent is not required to maintain records of the financial transactions or present the records to any third party representative. If the principal has become incapacitated and is not able to demand an accounting of the assets, the agent may exert extensive financial control over the principal's property and not have any accountability for the expenditures (Weiler, 1989).

Joint Tenancy Accounts

Another financial relationship that is very common for all adults is a bank account held in joint tenancy. When an account is opened at a financial institution, a form must be signed, and, usually, if the account is in the name of two or more persons, the form requires the parties to stipulate the legal relationship that the parties will have with regard to the money in the account. If the account is held as a joint tenancy, one party is not a substitute decision maker for the other party. All of the parties are coowners of the account. The owners of the joint tenancy account share in all the benefits and responsibilities of the account. In addition, upon the death of one coowner, the remainder of the account immediately shifts to the surviving party(ies) and becomes the property of the surviving coowner(s) (Krauskopf, Brown, & Tokarz, 1996).

This form of private bank account is frequently used by spouses or as a convenience account for nonspousal parties (e.g., adult child and older parent). With the joint tenancy account, both parties may deposit or withdraw from the account. The parties are not required to use the assets of the account for the benefit of each other, and upon the death of one party the account becomes the undisputed property of the surviving party (Krauskopf, Brown, & Tokarz, 1996).

A joint tenancy account has the advantages of: being a private financial arrangement: one co-owner may manage the account if the other co-owner is incapacitated; in a financial emergency, any co-owner has immediate access to the account; and upon the death of one co-owner, the assets of the account immediately shift to the surviving co-owner. The primary disadvantage of a joint tenancy account is that the co-owners have no obligation to use the assets of the account for the benefit of the other co-owner(s). Therefore, one co-owner may become incapacitated (parent), and the other co-owner(s) (child) may use the assets for his or her own benefit. The surviving co-owner (child) has no legal obligation to share the balance of the account with others not listed on the account (siblings) (Krauskopf, Brown, & Tokarz, 1996).

Trusts

The establishment of a trust offers the maximum opportunity to maintain control of financial assets while transferring the management responsibilities usually associated with the ownership of property. A trust is a written document with defined property to be managed in a specified manner by an identified party (trustee) for the benefit of specific party(ies), (beneficiaries) (e.g., parents, grandchildren). The structure of a trust may be tailored to meet the specific needs of the beneficiaries. However, all trusts contain the following elements: restrictions that apply only to the property held by the trust; a named representative who is required to follow the dictates of the trust; and requirements for record keeping of the transactions involving the trust property. The major disadvantage in establishing a trust is the long-term expense associated with maintaining the trust. The costs associated with the trust limit this financial planning option to individuals who have the financial resources to pay for the associated fees (Krauskopf, Brown, & Tokarz, 1993).

Autonomy in personal, financial, and health care treatment decisions is a valued ethical principle among American young, middle-aged and older adults. The presumption that an adult has the right to make his or her own decisions is the foundation for legal options that allow for future planning or court intervention if the adult lacks decision-making capacity. During periods of transition in various aspects of the adult's life, discussed previously, it is the high value that Americans place on individual autonomy that necessitates the legal mechanisms for extension of an adult's decision-making capacity. In addition to these legal mechanisms, there are mechanisms, based on the ethical principle of beneficence, that are available for the surrogate decision maker.

Beneficence

Beneficence has been explained as the duty to (1) prevent evil or harm; (2) remove evil or harm; 3) do or promote good (Beauchamp & Childress,1994). All of these actions are premised on the principle that one should act in ways that will prevent or reduce harm and will benefit others (Wicclair, 1991). Another characteristic of beneficence is to view each decision from the perspective of the health care recipient's "best interests" (Aiken & Catalano, 1994; Mouton, Johnson, & Cole, 1995). The opposite concept of beneficence is paternalism, and it occurs if health care providers assume that they know what the patient, who has retained some decision-making capacity, would want or would chose even if the patient has not been given an opportunity to participate in the decision-making process (Aiken & Catalano, 1994; Mouton et al., 1995). The assumption of the health care providers may coincide with the patient's assessment of his or her own best interests or may be directly opposite the patient's own wishes. The essential rule that applies to all health care treatment decisions is that the patient has the right to participate in the decision-making process to the maximum extent that he or she is able, or desires, to participate.

For adults who have diminished capacity or who lack decision-making capacity, there are several legal mechanisms that have been created so that a substitute or surrogate decision maker is empowered to make decisions in the incapacitated adult's "best interests." The terminology that each state uses may vary; however, each state has some system that gives the judicial system the authority to appoint a substitute or surrogate decision maker for a proposed ward, either a minor or incapacitated adult, so that the proposed ward's interests in personal, health care, and financial decisions will be protected (Smyer, Schaie, & Kapp, 1996).

For clarity of discussion, this chapter will limit the use of the term "guardian" to a person who is court appointed and authorized to make personal and health care treatment decisions for the ward, and a "conservator" will be identified as a court-appointed substitute decision-maker for the ward's financial decision making needs. In most states, an adult qualifies as needing a guardian if he or she is lacking in understanding or the capacity to make or carry out responsible decisions regarding his or her own care (Krauskopf, Brown, & Tokarz, 1996; Uniform Guardianship and Protective Proceedings Act, 1997).

The individual states cannot assume that all guardianship petitions are initiated with beneficent intentions; therefore, frequently the guardianship proceeding may involve the appointment of legal representation for the proposed ward and separate legal representation for the proposed guardian. With this system it is possible that the proceeding may become adversarial, even though both parties believe that they are honestly representing the best interests of the proposed ward. The purpose of the separate legal representation is to provide protection for the proposed ward's right of autonomy and self-determination. Separate legal representation is intended to specifically protect the proposed ward's interests and advocate for the ward in any way that he or she may not be able to advocate for his or her own care (Kapp, 1994; Krauskopf, Brown, & Tokarz, 1996).

A conservatorship is a court-authorized relationship in which the conservator assumes control of the ward's financial assets. As compared to the guardianship, this relationship is not designed to authorize substitute or surrogate decision making for personal or health care treatment decisions; rather, a conservatorship is intended to be limited to decisions regarding the ward's financial assets. The extent of authority that the conservator has over the ward's financial assets is designated by the court. The conservator also is responsible for filing a regular financial report with the court that indicates how the conservator has protected the ward's financial assets and how the assets have been dispersed to protect the ward's long-term or short-term financial needs (Krauskopf, Brown, & Tokarz, 1993).

Nonmaleficence

Nonmaleficence is the ethical value that identifies that individuals should not actively or passively allow harm to come to another person or specifically that nurses do not cause harm to their patients or allow others to harm the patients. Harm may be defined as physical harm, the infliction of pain or psychological harm, or depriving an individual of the freedom of opportunity or experiencing pleasure (Beauchamp & Childress,1994).

The legal mechanism created to support the ethical principal of non-maleficence is embodied in the legal statutes that prohibit elder mistreatment by a caregiver, family member, or acquaintance. Although statutes defining elder mistreatment exist in all 50 states, there are differences in both their definition and whether they are categorized as elder mistreatment legislation or as part of a more broadly constructed adult protective services legislation (Hunzeker, 1990).

Protective laws to safeguard elderly people during periods of transition, when they are most vulnerable, have been passed in all 50 states. The statutes may be categorized as elder-abuse statutes or adult protective services legislation. While all states have legislative protection for elderly people, the content of the legislation may vary regarding (1) the definition of who is protected by the statute; (2) what kind of behavior is described as abusive behavior; (3) which settings provide protection from potential abuse, e.g., institutional or home care; (4) whether nurses and other health care providers are mandatory or voluntary reporters of suspected abuse; (5) whether there is a penalty for health care providers if suspected abuse is not reported; (6) if there are protections from liability if the health care provider makes a good faith reporting of suspected abuse; (7) which agency has the responsibility to investigate suspected abuse; and (8) if there are criminal sanctions for the abuser if the suspected abuse is confirmed (Hall & Weiler, 1996).

Generally, mistreatment of older adults is defined in terms of acts of commission (intentional infliction of harm) or acts of omission (harm occurring through neglect) by a caretaker. While the definition of a caretaker may vary among states, a typical definition includes "a related or nonrelated person who has the responsibility for the protection, care or custody of a dependent adult as a result of assuming the responsibility voluntarily, or by contract, through employment, or by order of the court " (Iowa, 235B § 2(1), 1996). The literature describes seven types of caregiver-initiated elder mistreatment, including physical abuse and neglect, sexual abuse, psychological abuse and neglect, financial/material exploitation, and violation of personal rights (Fulmer, 1991; Hirst & Miller, 1986; Quinn & Tomita, 1986; Sengstock & Hwalek, 1985) (see also Table 8.1). Individual cases may exhibit characteristics of multiple types of mistreatment with varying degrees of severity and research has indicated that mistreatment of an elder is seldom an isolated incident with physical abuse and neglect reoccurring in up to 80% of cases (O'Malley, O'Malley, Everitt, & Sarson, 1984).

Physical neglect is the most laden with definitional issues related to its multiple underlying etiologies. The primary issue is whether it should be subdivided further into the categories of active neglect (purposeful withholding of necessities) and passive neglect (legitimate inability of the care provider to perform caregiving duties) based on the intent and capacities of the caregiver (Bristowe, 1989). Sociocultural ambiguity underlies questions related to the nature and extent of family caretaker duties owed to elderly persons as the term "neglect" implies a failure to fulfill an obligation (Lachs & Fulmer, 1993; Phillips, 1988). These problems have led some researchers to abandon traditional mistreatment definitions and to conceptualize the problem as inadequate care of elderly persons (Fulmer, 1987) or to propose that a caregiving paradigm be used to formulate intervention strategies (Phillips, 1988). However, during these periods of transition from self-care to a situation of care provided by family members, it may be more appropriate to focus on legal interventions to protect the elderly victims than on counseling and education for the perpetrator(s) (Phillips, 1988).

The incidence of elder mistreatment has been estimated to range from 4% (Block & Sinnott, 1979) to 10% (Fulmer, 1992; Lau & Kosberg, 1979) of the aged population, affecting between 700,000 and 2.5 million elderly persons each year (Fulmer, McMahon, Baer-Hines, & Forget, 1992; Iowa Department of Elder Affairs, 1992). The discrepancy in prevalence rates has been attributed to methodologic limitations, extrapolation of small samples of the total elderly population of the United States (Pillemer &

TABLE 8.1 Types of Elder Mistreatment

Type	Characteristics
Physical Abuse	Intentional infliction of physical harm or unreasonable confinement resulting in bodily injury, anguish, or pain; violent acts that are typically at variance with the history given of them; repeated patterns of physical injury that intensify over time.
Physical Neglect	Willful or negligent acts or omissions that deprive the elder of minimum food, shelter, clothing, supervision, physical or mental health care, or other care necessary to maintain life or health.
Sexual Abuse	Any form of involuntary sexual contact including incest, rape, molestation, prostitution, or participation in sexual acts; acts that are typically perpetrated through threats of force, coercion, or misrepresentation.
Psychological Abuse	Verbal assault by a caretaker that dehumanizes and causes mental anguish to the elder, including name calling, ridiculing, humiliating, threatening, or inducing fear of isolation or removal.
Psychological Neglect	Failure of the caretaker to satisfy the emotional or psychological needs of an elder, including isolating the elder or not providing social or cognitive stimulation.
Financial/Material Exploitation	The act or process of using or taking the material goods of an elder for personal or pecuniary gain without consent or authority or through the use of undue influence.
Violation of Personal Rights	Taking unlawful advantage of the legally guaranteed rights of the elder, including denied contracting, involuntary servitude, unnecessary guardianship, or misuse of professional authority.

Suitor, 1988) and lack of specificity in elder mistreatment definitions. As increased numbers of Americans age and join the elderly population, the incidence of elder mistreatment also is expected to increase.

In the first large-scale study of mistreatment in community dwelling older adults, physical violence emerged as the most widespread (Pillemer & Finkelhor, 1988); however, in a study of hospital-based elders, the referrals for neglect occurred at approximately five times the rate as those for physical abuse (Carr et al., 1986). A review of elder mistreatment reports found that financial exploitation was the most frequently reported abuse (49%), followed by emotional abuse (36%) and neglect (33%) (Neale, Hwalek, Goodrich, & Quinn, 1996). This is consistent with the findings of others who have noted that financial exploitation is a common type of elder mistreatment (Ogg & Bennett, 1992), particularly among those with dementia (Rowe, Davies, Baburaj, & Sinha, 1993). Although the spousal abuse aspect of elder abuse has not received much attention, several studies suggest that it is a major underlying factor (Pillemer & Finkelhor, 1988; Wolf, 1986).

The importance of early identification and intervention lies in its potential for reducing or preventing the occurrence of elder mistreatment. However, detection of elder mistreatment parallels the problems of other forms of family violence in that the victims often do not complain because of their perceived dependency on the perpetrator or because of their fears of reprisal or embarrassment. Additional barriers to detection include cognitive impairments affecting the older adult's memory or their ability to communicate and the confounding of age-related vulnerabilities with mistreatment symptoms in areas such as falls, dehydration, malnutrition, and drug toxicity (Haviland & O'Brian, 1989).

It is estimated that 80% of health care for elderly persons is being provided by family members (Baines & Oglesby, 1992), and it has been consistently reported that family caregivers are the primary perpetrators of elder mistreatment (Anetzberger, 1987; Baines & Oglesby, 1992; Council on Scientific Affairs, 1987; Fulmer & Cahill, 1984; Gelles & Cornell, 1982; Homer & Gilleard, 1990; Kosberg, 1988; Pillemer & Finkelhor, 1988; Pillemer & Finkelhor, 1989; Tomita, 1982; Wolf, 1990). While researchers have reported that in 86% of mistreatment cases, the abuser is a relative who lives with the older adult approximately 75% of the time and has cared for him or her an average of 9.5 years (O'Malley, Everitt, & O'Malley, 1983), the findings vary as to the nature of the perpetrator's relationship to the victim. Some studies have found the abuser is most likely the elder's adult child (Hirst & Miller, 1986; Mildenberger & Wessman, 1986), while others have reported the perpetrator is most often a spouse (Hagebock & Brandt, 1981; Pillemer & Finkelhor, 1988; Wolf, 1986).

Variables associated with elder mistreatment have been reported in the literature and can be classified into four separate domains, including socio-cultural, family, caretaker, and individual characteristics of the older adult. Stress arising from these domains may be situational, acute, or chronic in nature. However, it should be noted that there is no litmus test for elder mistreatment, only related risk factors whose identification provides the opportunity for preventive measures to be directed at stressful environments or interpersonal relationships.

Modern medical technology has dramatically increased life expectancy resulting in protracted periods of time during which elderly people are susceptible to physical and emotional disabilities and subsequently have greater dependency needs. Shorter hospital stays and early discharges of elderly patients often result in rushed, unplanned and unrealistic placement decisions that fail to consider the elderly person's need for complex physical care, the family's lack of experience in providing such care, and the family's lack of preparedness for the long-term consequence of caring for a family member (Boland & Sims, 1996; Sims, Boland, & O'Neill, 1992). An additional sociocultural factor is the trend toward smaller family size, which results in a decreasing pool of relatives to provide care for an expanding group of vulnerable older adults. Among elderly mistreatment victims referred to social services agencies, the majority are dependent and frail with multiple impairments, and it has been proposed that dependency is a major factor in their mistreatment.

Identified family risk factors include a lack of family support, isolation, economic pressures, history of family violence (Fulmer, 1989; Grafstrom, Nordberg, & Wimbald, 1992; Straus, Gelles, & Steinmetz, 1981), and being unaware or ineligible for government or community assistance programs. Characteristics of the at-risk family caregiver that have been reported include (1) being overwhelmed and stressed in the caregiver role; (2) continued financial dependency of the abuser on the elderly person; (3) history of substance abuse; (4) poor health or physical frailty; (5) unrealistic expectations; (6) lack of interest in the elderly person's needs; and (7) lack of empathy or concern for the older family member.

Characteristics placing the elderly person at risk for mistreatment include advanced age (> 75 years old), multiple health problems that decrease the older adult's ability to function without assistance, functional dependence, cognitive loss or dementia, substance abuse and overly demanding behavior by the older adults. The caregiver's and elderly person's behavior, attitudes, and history of the injury (including patterns of injuries) can offer valuable clues to the presence of elder mistreatment and provide direction for interventions that address the older adult's needs.

An important barrier to detection and intervention of elder mistreatment is the failure of health care professionals to either include it as a differential diagnosis or to report assessment findings that indicate mistreatment . Researchers who examined factors that influence clinicians' assessment and management of family violence reported that (1) elder mistreatment was not frequently suspected by any discipline; (2) that 75% of the professionals had not received any education on mistreatment of elderly persons; (3) that formal educational training in family violence significantly predicted the reporting of elder physical abuse; and (4) among clinicians whose practice included elderly persons, only 32% of nurses included reporting as an intervention they use (Tilden et al., 1994). Clinicians also are affected in their judgment of elder mistreatment by the severity of the situation, the personalities of the elderly person and caregiver, and the degree of effort that clinicians perceive the caregiver as expending (Phillips & Rempusheski, 1985).

While primary preventive interventions are directed at the general public to promote the elderly person's self-reliance, independence, and family functioning to prevent elder mistreatment, secondary preventive interventions are directed at individuals and groups at risk for elder mistreatment to promote the maximum functional and coping abilities of elderly persons and their caregivers, and tertiary preventive interventions are directed at elderly persons and their caregivers after mistreatment has occurred to protect the older adult and prevent the reincidence of elder mistreatment. The most difficult legal and ethical dilemmas arise in the treatment of elder mistreatment when the patient insists on continuing in a relationship or environment in which he or she is mistreated. This may place the clinician in conflict with the older adult; however, the clinician has an obligation to explain that the older adult need not remain in this situation and to describe the available alternatives (Lachs & Fulmer, 1993).

Researchers have provided useful algorithms for intervening in cases of elder mistreatment for competent and incompetent elders (O'Malley, Everitt, & O'Malley, 1983). If an elderly person is incompetent or suspected to be incompetent, case management may require petitioning the court for a guardian or conservator. The clinician has two important roles in this process, including rendering an opinion with regard to the elderly person's decision-making capacity, which may be used in court proceedings, and providing documentation of the mistreatment, which will ensure that the perpetrator does not become the substitute decision maker for the older adult (Lachs & Fulmer, 1993). As discussed previously, many guardianship and conservatorship petitions are sincerely sought for the elderly person's protection. However, the judicial system cannot assume that all petitions are in the elderly person's best interests. Therefore, the court must explore the older adult's need for a surrogate decision maker.

Justice

Justice is described in terms of fairness and an individual receiving what he or she deserves or has earned (Beauchamp & Childress,1994). Giving what has been earned or what is deserved means that all who earn a reward should receive the reward and those who have not earned the reward should not receive it. One of the principles of justice is that equals must be treated equally and that different cases should be treated differently (Beauchamp & Childress, 1994; Wicclair, 1991). This principle may not elicit controversy until the description or definitions of equals and differ- ent cases are presented. The perceptions of equality are affected by a per- son's background. Inherent in this discussion is the need to acknowledge the role that past changes have had on the current elders (e.g., the Depression, World War II, the baby boom generation). Specifically, should all individuals be treated the same in the allocation of health care resources? Should there be special circumstances that enhance an individ- ual's access to health care, e.g., loss of limb or vital organ due to wartime service, life-threatening situations, or circumstances that limit an individ- ual's access to health care, e.g., terminal illnesses and potential futility of care? Who decides and which equation is used to decide if justice has been achieved in the allocation of health care resources?

For elderly persons, the controversy regarding allocation of health care resources has been a significant issue. Several arguments in support of rationing health care based on the person's age have been proposed:

1. the older patients have an obligation to preserve health care resources for the young;
2. society has a greater obligation to provide health care for children than for the elderly people;
3. the withholding of care from the elderly patient is not prematurely causing death but allowing the natural progression of death; and
4. age-based rationing is a fair criterion because it affects all people equally (Zweibel, Cassel, & Karrison,1993).

Opponents of the age-based rationing of health care assert that:

1. the elderly population is a heterogeneous, not a homogenous, group and deserves individualized treatment;
2. health care treatment decisions should not be mandated according to an age criterion but in the context of the physician-patient relationship;
3. elderly people have a greater need for care based on increased risks for illness and disabilities and the greater need, not the age, should determine access to care;
4. age-based rationing disproportionately discriminates against women; and
5. there is no assurance that the savings achieved by not treating elderly persons will be expended to improve the health care for younger adults and children (Faden & German, 1994; Kuder & Roeder, 1995; Pinch & Parsons, 1993; Zweibel et al., 1993).

A recent question associated with the principle that equals must be treated equally and that different cases should receive different care arose in the context of physician-assisted suicide (*Vacco v Quill*, 1997). In the *Quill* case, three New York physicians asserted that the New York statute prohibiting physician-assisted suicide prohibited equal treatment of those who were terminally ill. The physicians asserted that there was an inequity between the treatment received by competent adults, with a terminal illness, receiving life-sustaining treatment and the treatment given to terminally ill competent adults not receiving life-sustaining treatment. The physicians asserted that those on life-sustaining treatment could hasten their death by refusing the life-sustaining treatment; however, those who did not require life-support could not hasten their death by requesting physician-prescribed drugs for self-administration (*Vacco v Quill*, 1997).

The United States Supreme Court (*Vacco v Quill*, 1997) determined that an inequity in care did not exist for those who were competent, terminally ill, and received or did not receive life-sustaining treatment. Rather, the Court described that all of the patients were given equal treatment under the New York statute, "*Everyone*, regardless of physical condition, is entitled, if competent, to refuse unwanted lifesaving medical treatment; *no one* is permitted to assist a suicide" (emphasis in original) (*Vacco v Quill*, 1997). The Court then detailed the legal history that supported the determination that refusal of care is not equal to assisted suicide (*Vacco v Quill*, 1997).

The issues associated with justice and allocation of health care for elderly persons has been a source of considerable concern, and it seems unlikely that a resolution to the problem will be rapidly forthcoming.

CONCLUSION

Americans assume that specific ethical principles underlie the rights and responsibilities of adulthood. Those ethical principles are autonomy, beneficence, nonmalificence, and justice. Based on these principles, legal interventions or policies have been formulated to ensure individuals that the rights are protected and the responsibilities are enforced. The transitions from young, to middle, to older adulthood present many positive changes for adults. However, accompanied by the rewards of aging, there also are challenges and potential crises that may have a dramatic effect on the adult's future.

This chapter has explored some of the problems that some adults have encountered in their transition into the elder years. The problems and potential interventions have been identified, and, it is hoped they will provide insight into the range of personal, financial, and health care issues that may arise for adults as they age. The goal of the authors has been to identify the basic ethical principles and the associated legal options that an elderly person or a caregiver could explore in anticipation of the need for future assistance or as options for various current concerns.

REFERENCES

Aiken, T. D. & Catalano, J. T. (1994). *Legal, ethical, and political issues in nursing*. Philadelphia: F.A. Davis.

Anetzberger, G. J. (1987). *The etiology of elder abuse by adult offspring.* Springfield, MA: Charles C. Thomas.

Baines, E., & Oglesby, M. (1992). The elderly as caregivers of the elderly. *Holistic Nurse Practitioner, 7*(4), 61–69.

Baumhover, L. A., Beall, S. C., & Pieroni, R. E. (1990). Elder abuse: An overview of social and medical indicators. *Journal of Health and Human Resources Administration, 12*(4), 414–433.

Beauchamp, T. L., & Childress, J.F. (1994). *Principles of biomedical ethics* (4th ed.). New York: Oxford University Press.

Block, M. R., & Sinnott, J. D. E. (1979). *The battered elder syndrome: An exploratory study.* College Park, MD: University of Maryland Center on Aging.

Boland, D., & Sims, S. (1996). Family care giving at home as a solitary journey. *Image, 26*(1), 55–58.

Brent, N. J. (1997). *Nurses and the law: A guide to principles and applications.* Philadelphia: W.B. Saunders.

Bristowe, E. (1989). Family mediated abuse of noninstitutionalized frail elderly men and women living in British Columbia. *Journal of Elder Abuse and Neglect, 1*(1), 45–64.

Brophy v New England Sinai Hospital., Inc., 497 N.E.2d 626 (Mass. 1986).

Carr, K., Dix, G., Fulmer, T., Kaulsh, B., Dravitz, L., Matlaw, J., Mayer, J., Minaher, K., Wetle, T., & Zarle, N. (1986). An elder abuse assessment team in acute hospital setting. *The Gerontologist, 35,* 115–118.

Choice in Dying. (1994). New York: The National Council for the Right to Die.

Council on Scientific Affairs. (1987). Elder abuse and neglect. *Journal of the American Medical Association, 257,* 966–971.

Cruzan v. Director, Missouri Department of Health (1990). 110 S. Ct. 2841.

Faden, R., & German, P.S., (1994). Quality of life: Considerations in geriatrics. *Clinics in Geriatric Medicine, 10*(3), 541–551.

Fulmer, T. T. (1987). *Inadequate care of the elderly: A health care perspective on abuse and neglect.* New York: Springer.

Fulmer, T. T. (1989). Mistreatment of elders. Assessment, diagnosis, and intervention. *Nursing Clinics of North America, 24*(3), 707–716.

Fulmer, T. T. (1991). Elder mistreatment: Progress in community detection and intervention. *Family and Community Health, 14*(2), 26–34.

Fulmer, T. (1992). Clinical outlook: Elder mistreatment assessment as a part of everyday practice. *Journal of Gerontological Nursing, 18*(3), 42–45.

Fulmer, T. T., & Cahill, V. M. (1984). Assessing elder abuse: A study. *Journal of Gerontological Nursing, 10*(12), 16–20.

Fulmer, T., McMahon, D., Baer-Hines, M., & Forget, B. (1992). Abuse, neglect, abandonment, violence, and exploitation: An analysis of all elderly patients seen in one emergency department during a six-month period. *Journal of Emergency Nursing, 18,* 505–510.

Gelles, R. J., & Cornell, C. P. (1982, July). Elder abuse: The status of current knowledge. *Family relations, 31,* 457–465.

Grafstrom, M., Nordberg, A., & Wimbald, B. (1993). Abuse is in the eye of the beholder: Reports by family members about abuse of demented persons in home care: A total population based study. *Scandinavian Journal of Social Medicine, 21*(4), 247–255.

Hagebock, H., & Brandt, K. (1981). *Characteristics of elder abuse.* Unpublished manuscript . University of Iowa Gerontological Center at Iowa City.

Hall, G. R., & Weiler, K. (1996). Elder abuse, neglect and mistreatment. In C. W.

Bradway (Ed.), *Nursing care of geriatric emergencies* (pp. 225–251). New York: Springer Publishing Co.

Hall, J. K. (1996). *Nursing ethics and law*. Philadelphia: W. B. Saunders.

Haviland, S., & O'Brian, J. (1989). Physical abuse and neglect of the elderly: Assessment and intervention. *Orthopaedic Nursing, 8*(4), 11–19.

Hirst, S., & Miller, J. (1986). The abused elderly. *Journal of Psychosocial Nursing, 24*(10), 28–34.

Hobbs, F. B., & Damon, B. L. (1996). Current population reports. Special studies. *65+ in the United States (p23-190)*. Washington, D.C.: U.S. Bureau of the Census. Department of Commerce.

Homer, A. C., & Gilleard, C. (1990). Abuse of elderly people by their carers. *British Medical Journal, 301*(6765), 1359–1362.

Hunzeker, D. (1990). *State legislative response to crimes against the elderly*. National Conference of State Legislatures. Denver, CO.

Iowa Code, Chapter 235B (1996).

Kapp, M. B. (1994). Ethical aspects of guardianship. *Clinics in Geriatric Medicine, 10*(3), 501–512.

Kosberg, J. I. (1988). Preventing elder abuse: Identification of high risk factors prior to placement decisions. *The Gerontologist, 28*(1), 43–50.

Kosberg, J., & Cairl, R. (1986). The cost of care index: A case management tool for screening informal care providers. *The Gerontologist, 26,* 273–278

Krauskopf, J. M., Brown, R. N., & Tokarz, K. L. (1993). *Elderlaw: Advocacy for the aging* (2nd ed.). St. Paul, MN: West.

Krauskopf, J. M., Brown, R. N., & Tokarz, K. L. (1996 Suppl.). *Elderlaw: Advocacy for the aging* (2nd ed.). St. Paul, MN: West.

Kuder, L. B., & Roeder, P. W. (1995). Attitudes toward age-based health care rationing. *Journal of Aging and Health, 7*(2), 301–327.

Lachs, M., & Fulmer, T. (1993). Recognizing elder abuse and neglect. *Clinics in Geriatric Medicine, 9,* 665–681.

Lau, E., & Kosberg, J. (1979). Abuse of the elderly by informal care providers. *Aging, 12,* 10–15.

Mappes, T. A., & Zembaty, J. A. (1986). *Biomedical ethics* (2nd ed.). New York: Mc-Graw-Hill.

Mildenberger, C., & Wessman, H. (1986). Abuse and neglect of elderly persons by family members. *Physical Therapy, 66*(4), 537–539.

Mouton, C. P., Johnson, M. S., & Cole D. R. (1995). Ethical considerations with African-American elders. *Clinics in Geriatric Medicine, 11*(1), 113–129.

Neale, A., Hwalek, M., Goodrich, C., & Quinn, K. (1996). The Illinois elder abuse system: Program description and administrative findings. *The Gerontologist, 36*(4), 502–511.

Northrop, C. E., & Kelly, M. E. (1987). *Legal issues in nursing*. St. Louis: C. V. Mosby.

Ogg, J., & Bennett, G. (1992). Elder abuse in Britain. *British Medical Journal, 305,* 998–999.

O'Malley, T.A., Everitt, D., O'Malley, H. & Campion, E. (1983). Identifying and preventing family mediated abuse and neglect of elderly persons. *Annals of Internal Medicine, 98*, 998–1005.

O'Malley, T. A., O'Malley, H. C., Everitt, D. E., & Sarson, D. (1984). Categories of family-mediated abuse and neglect of elderly persons. *Journal of American Geriatrics, 32*(5), 362–369.

Patient Self-Determination Act (PSDA) (1990). (Public Law 101-508), codified at 42 U.S.C.A. §§ 1395cc(a)(1)(Q), 1395mm c(8), 1395(f); 42 U.S.C.A. §§ 1396a(a)(57), (58), 1396a(w).

Phillips, L. R. (1988). The fit of elder abuse with the family violence paradigm, and the implications of a paradigm shift for clinical practice. *Public Health Nursing, 5*(4), 222–229.

Phillips, L. R., & Rempusheski, V. F. (1985). A decision-making model for diagnosing and intervening in elder abuse and neglect. *Nursing Research, 34*(3), 134–139.

Pillemer, K., & Finkelhor, D. (1988). The prevalence of elder abuse: A random sample survey. *The Gerontologist, 28*(1), 51–57.

Pillemer, K., & Finkelhor, D. (1989). Causes of elder abuse: Caregiver stress versus problem relatives. *American Journal of Orthopsychiatry, 59*(2), 179–187.

Pillemer, K., & Suitor, J. J. (1988). Elder abuse. In V. B. Van Hasselt (Ed.), *Handbook of family violence* (pp. 247–270). New York: Plenum Press.

Pinch, W. J., & Parsons, M. E. (1993). The ethics of treatment decision making: The elderly patient's perspective. *Geriatric Nursing, 14*(6), 289–293.

Quinn, M. J., & Tomita, S. K. (1986). *Elder abuse and neglect: Causes, diagnosis and intervention strategies.* New York: Springer.

Rowe, J., Davies, K., Baburaj, V., & Sinha, R. (1993). F.A.D.E.A.W.A.Y: The financial affairs of dementing elders and who is the attorney. *Journal of Elder Abuse and Neglect, 5*(2), 73–79.

Schloendorff v. Society of New York Hospital. (1914). 211 N.Y. 125, 105 N.E. 92.

Schuster, M. (1996). In B. J. Collins (Ed.), *Elder law institute.* New York: Practising Law Institute.

Sengstock, M., & Hwalek, M. (1985). *Comprehensive index of elder abuse* (2nd ed.). Detroit, MI: SPEC Associates.

Sims, S. L., Boland, D. L., & O'Neill, C. (1992). Decision making in home health care. *Western Journal of Nursing Research, 14*, 186–200.

Smyer, M., Schaie, K. W., & Kapp, M. B. (1996). *Older adults' decision-making and the law.* New York: Springer.

Steinmetz, S. K. (1990). Elder abuse by adult offspring: The relationship of actual vs. perceived dependency. *Journal of Health and Human Resources Administration, 12*(4), 434–463.

Stephens, M. A. P., & Zarit, S. H. (1989). Symposium: Family caregiving to dependent older adults: Stress, appraisal, and coping. *Psychology and Aging, 4*(4), 387–388.

Straus, M., Gelles, R., & Steinmetz, S. (1981). *Behind closed doors: Violence in the American family*. New York: Doubleday.

Strauss P. J., & Lederman, N. M. (1996). *The elder law handbook: A legal and financial survival guide for caregivers and seniors*. New York: Facts On File.

Teno, J. M., Licks, S., Lynn, J., Wenger, N., Connors, A. F. Jr., Phillips, R. S., O'Connor, M. A., Murphy, D. P., Fulkerson, W. J., Desbiens, N., & Knaus, W. A. (1997). Do advance directives provide instructions that direct care? *Journal of the American Geriatrics Society, 45*(4), 508–512.

Tilden, V., Schmidt, T., Limandri, B., Chiodo, G., Garland, M., & Loveless, P. (1994). Factors that influence clinician's assessment and management of family violence. *American Journal of Public Health, 84*(4), 628–633.

Tomita, S. K. (1982). Detection and treatment of elderly abuse and neglect: A protocol for health care professionals. *Physical and Occupational Therapy in Geriatrics*, (2), 37–51.

Uniform Guardianship and Protective Proceedings Act (U.L.A.). (1997). St. Paul, MN: West Group.

Uniform Rights of the Terminally Ill Act (U.L.A.). (1985). St. Paul, MN: West Group.

U.S. Congress, Office of Technology Assessment. (1987, July). *Life-sustaining technologies and the elderly* (Ota-BA-306) Washington, DC: U.S. Government Printing Office.

Vacco v Quill, (1997), 65 U.S.L.W. 4695–4705.

Weiler, K. (1989). Financial abuse of the elderly: Recognizing and acting on it. *Journal of Gerontological Nursing 15*(8), 10–15.

Wicclair, M. R. (1991). Differentiating ethical decisions from clinical standards. *Dimensions of Critical Care Nursing, 10*(5), 280–288.

Willis, S.L. (1996). Assessing everyday competence in the cognitively challenged elderly. In M. Smyer, K. W. Schaie, & M. B. Kapp (Eds.), *Older adults' decision-making and the law*. New York: Springer.

Wolf, R. (1986). *Major findings from three model projects on elder abuse*. Dover, MA: Auburn House.

Wolf, R. S. (1990). Elder abuse: Scope, characteristics, and treatment. *Nurse Practitioner Forum, 1*(2), 102–108.

Zweibel, N. R., Cassel, C. K., & Karrison, T. (1993). Public attitudes about the use of chronological age as a criterion for allocating health care resources. *The Gerontologist, 33*(1), 74–80.

Index

('i' indicates an illustration, 't' indicates a table)

177

Springer Publishing Company

Nurse-Physician Collaboration
Care of Adults and the Elderly

Eugenia L. Siegler, MD, and
Fay W. Whitney, PhD, RN, FAAN, Editors

Foreword by **Joan Lynaugh and Barbara Bates**

Written by an RN-MD team, this book describes the current barriers to effective collaboration between nurses and physicians and suggests how to overcome them. Six successful examples of collaborative practice in a variety of settings are described. Specific guidelines for teaching collaborative skills to both physicians and nurses are outlined at length.

Today's health care trends are moving toward expanded use of nurse practitioners and other nurses with advanced training. In these circumstances, successful collaboration can mean better health care delivery for all.

Contents:

Springer Series on Advanced Nursing Practice
1994   264pp   0-8261-8500-2   hardcover

536 Broadway, New York, NY 10012-3955 • (212) 431-4370 • Fax (212) 941-7842

SP *Springer Publishing Company*

Restraint-Free Care
A Guide for Individualized Clinical Practice

Neville E. Strumpf, PhD, RN, C, FAAN
Joanne E. Patterson, PhD, RN
Joan Stockman Wagner, MSN, CRNP
Lois K. Evans, DNSc, RN, FAAN

This book is for individuals seeking information on restraint-free care. Organized in outline format, the authors highlight critical material to be readily adaptable as a quick reference for clinicians, or as an adjunct for teaching staff, educating administrators, board members, and consumers.

A philosophy of individualized care is the framework for this guide, which the authors believe to be key to understanding older adults and to providing restraint-free care. The goals of individualized care include promoting comfort and safety, optimizing function and independence, and achieving the greatest possible quality of life. Such care requires clinicians to make sense of behavior rather than to control responses of clients.

The book contains specific strategies of understanding behavior; effecting change for the individual, the environment and institution; managing the risk of falls; and interference with recent treatments. Case studies and lists of resources are included in this practical and information-packed resource.

Contents:

Preface • Rethinking Restraint Use • Implementing a Process of Change • Making Sense of Behavior • Responding to Behavioral Phenomena • Assessment and Prevention of Falls and Injurious Falls • Caring for the Person Who Interferes with Treatment • Maintaining a Process of Change

1998   168pp   0-8261-1215-3   softcover

536 Broadway, New York, NY 10012-3955 • (212) 431-4370 • Fax (212) 941-7842